I Remember Better When I Paint

Art and Alzheimer's:
Opening Doors, Making Connections

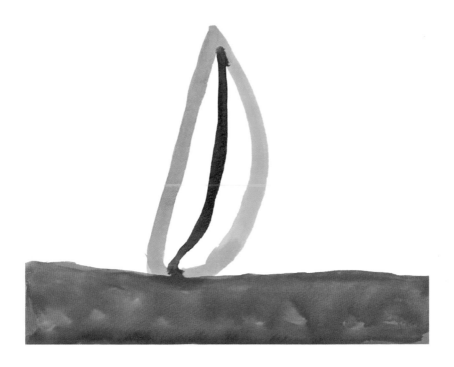

Berna G. Huebner
Editor

Bethesda Communications Group
and New Publishing Partners

Published by the Bethesda Communications Group
   and New Publishing Partners
49 Wellesley Circle, Glen Echo, MD 20812
www.bcgpub.com

ISBN 978-0-9761364-4-6

Cover design by Jenny Graf Sheppard and Deborah Lange

Book design, image editing, and text editing by Deborah Lange

Image selection by Jenny Graf Sheppard, Inge-Lise Sheppard, and Deborah Lange

The Hilgos Foundation wishes to thank the following for permission to reprint their works of art:

   Galerie Beckel Odille Boîcos, 1, rue Jacques Coeur, 75004 Paris — paintings
      by William Utermohlen on page 40
   Solomon R. Guggenheim Museum, New York — ...Whose Name Was Writ
      in Water (1975) by Willem de Kooning on page 41
   Hirshhorn Museum and Sculpture Garden, Smithsonian Institution, Holenia
      Purchase Fund, in Memory of Joseph H. Hirshhorn, 1991. Photography by
      Lee Stalsworth. — Untitled (1985) by Willem de Kooning on page 41
   Joeen Rodinsky — photograph on page 55
   Jenny Graf Sheppard — photograph on page 73
   Timothy Daly — drawings on pages 77 and 87
   Robin Barcus-Slonina — drawing on page 98

All other paintings and photographs are from the Hilgos Foundation Collection.

All proceeds from the sale of this book go to support programs that promote artistic projects and research activities for people who have Alzheimer's disease or other diseases that impair memory.

Contents

Expanded Contents

Part I: The Intersection of Medicine, Art, and Creative Therapies

1. **The Creative Arts and Alzheimer's: New Insights, New Possibilities**
   Robert N. Butler, M.D.

   Founder of the National Institute on Aging, the Alzheimer's Association, and the International Longevity Center, Dr. Butler writes that experience with Alzheimer's patients has shown that positive attitudes and consistent engagement by caregivers can re-establish communication between patients and the people in their environment. Dr. Butler concludes that engaging the patient in a rewarding activity–for example, an arts program– creates a wellness orientation that helps patients gain back their identities.

2. **Creativity and Art in Promoting Health and Coping with Alzheimer's**
   Gene D. Cohen, M.D., Ph.D.

   A pioneer in the field of geriatric psychiatry, Dr. Cohen states: *The Creativity and Aging Study* has shown that creatively engaging older adults in artistic activity improves their general and mental health and social activity. The underlying mechanisms are a sense of control and social engagement, which enhance the immune system. In addition, two helpful activities are the *Video Biography*, in which family members obtain stories that reflect happy or interesting life events, and the board game *Making Memories Together*, which uses

Memory Cards that have pictures and text drawn from four categories: places and special events, people, animals, and favorite objects. These activities offer many benefits, including positive shared experiences, better intergenerational family relations, and improved staff perception of the patient. They help strengthen connections between persons with Alzheimer's and their families and caregivers.

3. Art and the Brain
Avertano Noronha, M.B.B.S., M.D.

Neurologist Avertano Noronha notes that because the artist Hilgos showed a remarkable improvement in well-being after she returned to painting, we have two areas worth researching: (1) looking at strategies to encourage artistic activity in individuals with cognitive impairment, and (2) examining the effects of impairment on artistic expression. A benefit of the creative activity to all individuals is that it stimulates the brain and gives the individual a sense of accomplishment. It reduces depression and feelings of isolation. Physical exercise and exposure to novel stimuli are also shown to induce the brain to create new neurons, leading to improved cognitive function. As for the effects of impairment, Alzheimer's disease (AD) and Frontotemporal dementia (FTD) have different effects. AD causes progressive memory loss. FTD affects inhibitions and can cause changes in personality and impairment in planning and social functioning. Among the well-known artists and musicians who suffered from these diseases, we can determine which disease each one had by looking at their artistic creations.

4. Restoring the Sense of Self: Hilgos's Story
Lawrence W. Lazarus, M.D., D.F.L.A.P.A

Dr. Lazarus, Past-President of the American Association for Geriatric Psychiatry and the geriatric psychiatrist who suggested enlisting art students to work with Hilda, notes that the restoration of a patient's sense of self and a comprehensive evaluation and treatment plan are essential elements of patient care. Nursing staff members need to understand who the patient was. Family members can provide memorabilia, such as photographs and trophies, to help educate the staff. Staff can be taught conversational techniques for empathizing with and engaging a patient. Patients often retain musical and artistic skills learned early in life, which offer opportunities for working with the patient. A thorough evaluation of the patient can identify treatable medical problems, such as vitamin deficiency and depression. Understanding the patient's cultural background and providing support to family caregivers are also important to an effective the treatment plan.

Part II: The Artists' Stories

5. Revelation and Legacy
Berna G. Huebner

Berna Huebner, daughter of the artist Hilda Gorenstein, gives a personal view of her mother. She describes her mother's early interest in art and her career as a marine painter. She also shows how a love of beauty in art and nature infused her mother's spirit and informed her daily activities. When Hilda developed Alzheimer's and was moved to a nursing home, she became withdrawn and passive. She began to blossom, however, when students from the School of the Art Institute of Chicago started painting with her. Eventually Hilda regained speech, exhibited her work in an art show, and enjoyed other creative activities.

6. The Hidden Hour
Jenny Graf Sheppard

The first of four art students to work with artist Hilda Gorenstein, Jenny Graf Sheppard recounts the rewards and challenges of her experience. She writes: I was beginning my studies at the School of the Art Institute of Chicago when I accepted a job to paint three days a week with Hilda. She was initially unresponsive when I set up a table for painting, painted some strokes, and tried to hand off the brush to her. Eventually, however, as I let myself become her student, following her lead, she participated more. And then one day she worked alone without handing the brush back to me and completed a painting she named *The Hidden Hour*. Many setbacks followed that event. By the end of the year, however, three other artists had joined me and as a group we witnessed Hilda emerge from her shell and grow to a place where she would freely articulate thoughts.

7. The Invincible Circle
Timothy Daly

The second art student to join the group, Timothy Daly, writes: Visual communication through art gave Hilda a steady focus and let her say what she needed to say, both verbally and visually. I came to treasure the daily two hours I spent with her, and it was always a treat to see her face light up when I entered the room. After I visited her house and became familiar with her earlier sculptures and other works, I understood her graceful, poetic movements and connected with her interest in the horizon and ocean life. She also liked museum trips, where she could experience and discuss the paintings of others. Hilda taught me many things, especially how important patience is to the artistic process.

8. Hitting a Different Spot
Jane Benson

The third art student to join the group, Jane Benson, writes: Hilda found inspiration for her paintings in the photographs and postcards that her daughter Berna sent her. She often started painting directly onto a postcard or photograph, creating beautiful and complex images and enmeshing the real and the representational into a multi-layered relationship. Her own reality appeared to those around her to be a representation of reality, one filtered, obscured, and complicated by a mind that could morph memory and a conventional sense of things. As I guided Hilda's thoughts and gentle hand toward blank paper, there would be a transition in her mood. She spent longer on these paintings and grew calmer during their production. Completion would bring a sense of clarity and peace.

9. Hilda: A Jewel Distilled
Robin Barcus-Slonina

The fourth art student to join the group, Robin Barcus-Slonina, writes: By the time I began working with Hilda, Jenny Sheppard, Tim Daly, and Jane Benson had laid the groundwork. All I needed to do was ask, "Do you want to paint?" and the answer was invariably yes. With her materials placed in front of her, the transformation in her face and eyes was phenomenal, as she expertly began to paint. Color choices reflected her mood, and her most prevalent theme was nautical, as it had been for most of her life. Following the classic pattern of many great artists, her work had become more abstract than her earlier paintings. At times she became so relaxed while painting that she fell asleep and would resume her painting on awakening. I often sketched her during her catnaps, and an associate of hers, on seeing my drawings, was stunned to learn that I had known Hilda only briefly. He had felt my drawings had captured her earlier self. However, our artist group did not see in Hilda what was lost, but saw rather a creative, strong woman whose spirituality was punctuated by flashes of spunk, drive, ironic humor, and a sharp intellect.

Part III: Using Art and Creative Therapies

10. The Lessons of My Journey
Berna G. Huebner

Berna Huebner highlights the knowledge gained by artists, cognitive scientists, and physicians, and calls for more interdisciplinary work between the people in these fields so that all people with Alzheimer's can benefit from the most recent advances in knowledge about brain activity. She also recommends specific steps for Alzheimer's patients, their families, and their caregivers to help the patients regain and retain memories.

11. Now What? Including Art in Caring for Patients With Memory Loss
Dorothy Seman, R.N., M.S.

Dorothy Seman, former Coordinator of Home and Community-Based Programs at the Jesse Brown VA Medical Center, suggests ways of caring for persons with dementia and calls for friends and family members to help educate the community. She explains why art is meaningful to persons with memory loss, describes the variety of settings in which art can be part of the care plan, and tells what to expect when working with a person who has dementia. She also addresses the need to educate physicians, other health care professionals, and the general community on ways to help individuals with memory loss live their lives fully, and offers several methods for doing so.

12. Additional Comments from Doctors and Caregivers
Deborah Lange

Deborah Lange selects passages from the documentary film *I Remember Better When I Paint* that comment on the science of Alzheimer's disease, the effect on the individual, the effect of creative activities, and the state of Alzheimer's care today.

13. References and Resources: Assistance for Alzheimer's Patients, Their Families, and Their Caregivers
Dorothy Seman, R.N., M.S. and Berna G. Huebner

Dorothy Seman and Berna Huebner list websites, books, games, films, and recent research that can help people with Alzheimer's disease.

Acknowledgments

During the writing of *I Remember Better When I Paint* and the filming of its documentary companion of the same name, hundreds of friends and associates have contributed to my journey to understand better the intersection of art, medicine, and science in the lives of people with Alzheimer's disease and other forms of dementia.

Alzheimer's has become a global epidemic, and the search for a preventative or curative breakthrough is understandably a critical priority. At the same time, however, it is also crucial that we not neglect the many millions of people who already have Alzheimer's today or those who will be touched by it in the years immediately ahead. The evidence is growing rapidly that the creative arts can bring a new sense of identity, peace and joy to those who are afflicted by Alzheimer's, turning "victimization into victory" in the words of my friend, the art historian Roberta Gray Katz.

I would like to thank some of those whose efforts were so important in the creation of this book. First, my mother, whose words provided the title and whose example is the inspiration for this project. Next my family: Lee, Charley, and David Huebner. Also my father, Ed Gorenstein, my brother Leo Gorenstein, and his family, Sue Carrell and Danny Gorenstein, as well as Wendy and John Huebner.

The guiding lights for this project include, very importantly, my mother's doctor, Lawrence Lazarus, MD, and the art students from the School of the Art Institute of Chicago who worked with her: Jenny Sheppard, Jane Benson, Tim Daly and Robin Barcus-Slonina. They were guiding lights for us. I would also like to thank most warmly Jenny's mother, Inge-Lise Sheppard, and Jenny's godmother, Deborah Lange, the publisher and designer of this book. Frank Samuel has my special appreciation for helping to bring this project to fruition. I would also like to thank Audrey Wolf for her help with this project and Cathy Nolan, Pat Lair, and Tijana Maneva for their assistance.

My thanks also go to the School of the Art Institute of Chicago, its chancellor and former president Tony Jones, the former dean Carol Becker, Robyn Guest, Nancy Crouch, Randy Vick, Cathy Moon, James Allen, and Nancy and Ed Paschke.

Others who have been instrumental in advancing this project, and to whom I am most deeply grateful, are Sandy and Charles Incorvia, Charles Nolan, Robert Green, and all of those whose written accounts appear in this book.

This project would not have been possible without the dedication of the entire Hilgos team. And, at risk of omitting other deserving friends, I would mention the valued contributions of Mary Louise Stott, Susan Firestone Hahn, Susannah Goodman, Lee Goff, Kitty deZwart, Jinny Ewald, Anne Boylan, Nancy Kissinger, Jo Minow, Mary Lou and Norb Gold, Joeen Rodinsky, Irma and Harvey Keller, Julie Gottlieb, Nancy Visenberg, Sarah Lee Schupf, Helen Royland, Johnnie Jones, Franny Zorn, Ann Thayer, Sue Hine, Penny Rotheiser, Mary and Clarke Caywood, Kai Romero, Sally Bell, Anne Ryan, Angie Levenstein, Marilyn Glazer, Nancy Paul, Phoebe Goldman, Sandy Ellis-Grannis, Claire Weiler, Margot Levin Schiff, Betty Friedan, Catherine O'Neill, Richard Reeves, Mary and Paul Anderson, Heather Burns, Marianne Lester, Vivian Cruise, Anna Lascar, Marcia Gordon, Anne–Marie and Gene Marans, Myrna Lewis and Jacqueline Samuel.

Finally, it is in memory of my mother, called Hillie by her family, that we present this book to you, using her simple but profound words, "I Remember Better When I Paint."

Berna Huebner
August 2011

Foreword

Robert C. Green, M.D., M.P.H.

As a clinical researcher in Alzheimer's disease, I am thrilled by the progress that has taken place over the past ten years. We have symptomatic treatments available that are improving the lives of patients. There are compounds in clinical trials today that have the potential to slow or even prevent the disease altogether.

But as a practicing neurologist who sits with patients and their families each and every day, I am deeply saddened as I watch the agonies of people who are losing their cognitive abilities and the families suffering with them.

Alzheimer's disease is still an illness with many mysteries. In particular, we cannot look inside the minds of patients who have the disease and know what is lost and what is still there. But we do have hints that remarkable pools of knowledge and understanding are preserved even when the disease has progressed into moderate or late stages. I am regularly told by families that a patient will respond to a random question in a way that reflects surprising understanding. Sometimes, even a patient that has been mute will make a statement or respond to something overheard with surprising alacrity.

Families and professional caregivers realize that there is often more substance hidden within the mind of an Alzheimer's patient than can be measured. Programs of mental stimulation such as "reminiscence"[1] are recommended within the homes of community dwelling patients and are now standard in special care units for patients with Alzheimer's disease.

What we learn in this book is inspiring and, more importantly, useful for families all over the world who are struggling with this

---

1   The Reminiscence Program involve reaching the memories residing in the still viable regions of the brain by using music, pictures, and other aids.

disease. The painter known as Hilgos lost her abilities to remember, to recognize loved ones and even to speak. And yet with the loving attention of her family and art students, she picked up a paint brush again and produced surprisingly sophisticated paintings. The resurgence of her painting was unequivocally a source of pleasure to her and a source of joy to her family and friends. Without a doubt, it improved the quality of life for all involved.

The lesson of this book for families struggling with Alzheimer's disease is clear: even in the midst of decline, there is hope for connection. Even in the midst of silence, there are ways to speak across the void. The story of Hilgos is a reminder for us all and an inspiration for families everywhere.

Dr. Robert C. Green is Associate Director for Research, Partners Center for Genetic Medicine, Brigham and Women's Hospital and Harvard Medical School.

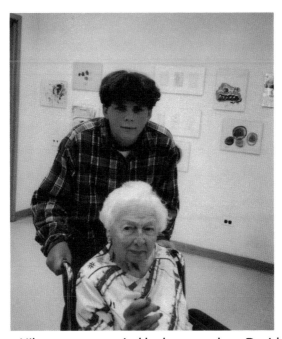

The painter Hilgos, accompanied by her grandson David Huebner, enjoys a gallery showing of her recent paintings..

Introduction

Searching for Connection: My Journey Begins

Berna G. Huebner

"Your mother has no mind. She cannot talk. She cannot understand. She is void." That was how I interpreted the reaction of nursing home staff and doctors when I suggested that my mother wanted to paint again. "Alzheimer's," they said. "You said she wanted to paint, but it's no use working with her."

I was despondent. My mother, who had once been so lively, so inspirational and such a renowned professional painter and sculptor, was a shell of her former self. She had quickly slipped into the somnambulant state of so many people afflicted with

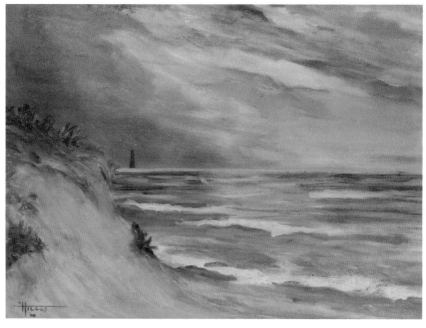

The Old Ludington Light, painted by Hilgos in 1938

Alzheimer's. However, even in my despair, I couldn't believe that it would be "no use working with her." And I couldn't stop turning over in my mind something my mother had told me earlier. As she struggled with memory loss in her later years, I had asked her if she wanted to paint. And she had said most definitely, "Oh yes! I remember better when I paint."

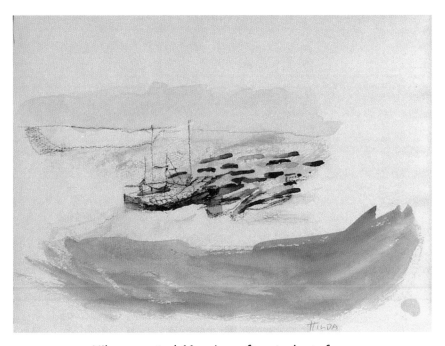

Hilgos created *Moorings* after students from
the Art Institute encouraged her to resume painting.

With that phrase ringing in my mind, I became determined to bring my mother back from her detached state. And so I enlisted the help of her psychiatrist, Dr. Lawrence Lazarus from Rush Presbyterian St. Luke's Medical Center in Chicago, the one physician who agreed with me that art therapy might work with my mother. With the miraculous, patient work of Dr. Lazarus, dedicated art students, and her family, my mother, Hilda Gorenstein (artist name Hilgos), picked up a brush and at age 91 began to paint again. Through painting and sculpting, she emerged from her listless state and reconnected to the world around her.

She reflected that world through art and painting. Her art student companions enjoyed taking her to the Art Institute of Chicago and other Chicago museums where she experienced again the masterpieces she had studied and loved all her life. As a result of all this, she spoke, she danced, she played catch, she sculpted. And she painted and painted and painted.

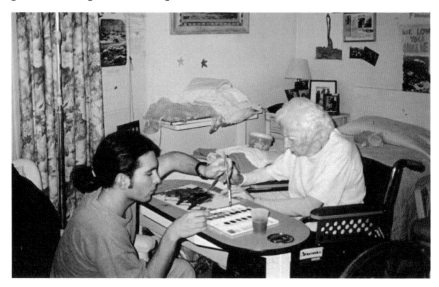

Hilgos and her grandson Charley Huebner enjoy painting together.

The essays by art students who worked with my mother tell the story of how my mother stopped withdrawing, began to live again, and rejoined our lives. And the chapters by physicians and a nurse help place her story in context and guide families seeking to make comparable connections with their loved ones.

Berna Huebner, Hilda Gorenstein's daughter, is founder and president of The Hilgos Foundation and co-director of the documentary "I Remember Better When I Paint." At the School of the Art Institute of Chicago, she originated the Hilgos Award for students working with people with memory loss. She is on the Board of Directors for the Center for the Study of International Communications in Paris, France. She is the former Research Director for Nelson Rockefeller when he was Governor of New York and then Vice President.

Part I: The Intersection of Medicine, Art, and Creative Therapies

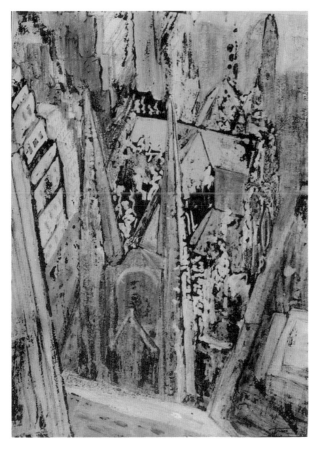

St. Patrick's Cathedral by Hilgos, 1969

1 The Creative Arts and Alzheimer's: New Insights, New Possibilities

Robert N. Butler, M.D.

Programs that bring people together and enrich each other's lives through the creative arts are a key to better Alzheimer's care.

Throughout my professional career, I have time and again been brought face to face with the twin features of our increased longevity: benefits and challenges. Indeed these two features are so intrinsic to our longer lives that I made them the subtitle of my most recent book, *The Longevity Revolution: The Benefits and Challenges of Living a Long Life.*[1]

Persons with Alzheimer's disease and their families and caregivers are only too aware of the challenges of this disease. And they have a lot of company. Consider the following data from the Alzheimer's Study Group's recent report.[2]

- 5 million people are afflicted with Alzheimer's disease in the U.S.

- Alzheimer's disease is the sixth leading cause of death.

- Alzheimer's disease affects the family, not just the afflicted person, with 10 million caregivers providing 94 billion (yes, billion!) hours of uncompensated care yearly.

---

1 Butler M. D., Robert N. *The Longevity Revolution: The Benefits and Challenges of Living a Long Life.* New York: Public Affairs, Perseus Books Group, 2008.

2 Gingrich, Newt and Bob Kerrey, Co-Chairs. *A National Alzheimer's Strategic Plan: The Report of the Alzheimer's Study Group.* (http://www.alz.org/documents/national/report_ASG_alzplan.pdf). 2009. (In 2010 the number of people rose to 5.3 million.)

- It is the third most expensive disease, costing the Federal government alone more than $100 billion annually.

And, as if these numbers weren't arresting enough, Alzheimer's disease is expected to increase by 50% in the next 20 years.

Yes, the challenges of Alzheimer's disease for families and our nation are only too obvious.

Where among all the challenges, one may ask, can anybody find a benefit? Surely benefits of this disease are non-existent. Surely the physical decline, the daily frustration, the bleak outlook conspire to make the challenges of this particular aging disease all-consuming and the suggestion of any benefit a cynical illusion.

Indeed, it is quite true that improvements like suppression of symptoms and reversal of decline must await further basic and applied research and the preventive techniques and new therapies that will result from new knowledge.

In the meantime, is there anything to do except wring our hands and do our best to keep a stiff upper lip while coping with the repetitive, apparently unrewarding conditions that greet 5 million of us when we look in our own mirrors or when many of us visit our family members and friends in nursing homes and hospitals?

The chapters that follow offer a powerful positive answer to this question. In most respects, Hilda Gorenstein, an accomplished Chicago artist known as Hilgos, was a typical Alzheimer's sufferer. She lost memory and the ability to function in daily life, she was confined to a nursing home surrounded by others like her and by unimaginative professionals, and she faced a future of further decline, frustration, and despair.

But the people who cared about her were able to make that future different. These were, initially, her family, and later, four art students from the School of the Art Institute of Chicago. All started out as ordinary helpers: a daughter, a son, and students. All ended up having remarkably positive influences on Hilda's quality of life and changing their own perceptions of what is possible. In Dr. Robert Green's words, they proved that "there is hope for connection."

Learning about Hilda's experience will help us to think of Alzheimer's in a new way. In the moments when she painted, she lived. With the help of the visiting art students, Hilgos made more than 300 paintings. As her doctor, Lawrence Lazarus, observed, the painting activity restored her self-esteem, overall functioning, and mood.

One aspect of Hilda's situation may, at first glance, appear to differentiate her from the growing multitude of persons with Alzheimer's and other forms of memory loss: her life-long activity as a painter. This provided an obvious tool to use in attempting—successfully, as it turned out—to re-engage Hilda in a rewarding activity.

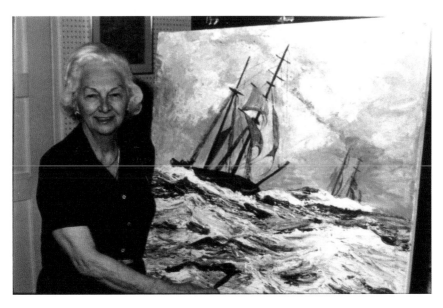

Hilgos with one of her marine paintings.

Of course, not all persons with memory loss are accomplished painters. Only a few might consider themselves accomplished in anything outside of their daily occupations, now irretrievably lost. Being able to rely on past achievements may appear to be available to only a very small percentage of those afflicted with Alzheimer's disease.

But such a view of what is possible is too narrow. From my decades of research and observation of aging and of specific disease states associated with it, I have become convinced that positive attitudes and consistent engagement on the part of caregivers are more important than the presence or absence of a particular activity in a person's history. Hilda's art students approached their shared activity—painting in her case—with a positive, engaged attitude that they maintained over the last years of her life. Painting was the tool; attitude and engagement made up the environment in which the tool's potential could be brought to fruition. I believe that comparable tools are available from the lives of most people.

And you will see powerful evidence that one of the benefits from Hilda's interacting with her family and the art students as she resumed painting was the sense of connection that was eventually re-established between Hilda, her family, and the four art students who visited and worked with her. These connections came only after a struggle. But the same is true of teaching youngsters to paint, play the piano, or persevere with soccer.

Hilda's ability to re-engage in painting and to teach art as she did lives on in these pages. It provides a powerful example as we begin to explore how creativity offers expression to a person with Alzheimer's who is losing verbal communication and a grasp of the world around her. Painting can provide insight into the current environment as perceived by this person at *this* moment. It can allow memories to be shared when language is gone. Hilda's story is a vivid affirmation that the arts can transcend illness and celebrate humanness.

The truth of this principle is vividly reported in the student essays later in this book. Despite frustrations and obstacles, the students developed a special relationship with Hilda, communicating largely through the artistic process they shared. One student said that by far the biggest lesson she learned working with Hilda was that the creative process is as essential to an artist as breathing, especially after it has been cultivated over the course of a lifetime.

As the students' collaboration with her progressed, they made another important discovery. They discovered, as they say forcefully, that the relationship they developed was a two-way street. They were not only helping an elderly artist with her painting, but also learning from her, developing new insights into their own lives, and into the meaning of the artistic process. Their experience confirms the validity of Dr. Robert Green's conclusion that there is hope for new connections between persons afflicted with Alzheimer's and their caregivers.

These student essays tell a story about a *wellness* orientation for an Alzheimer's patient. It is about an artist titling her exhibitions and signing her paintings. It is about a woman who danced, sculpted, and painted. It is about the focus of such an artist and about gaining back identity instead of losing it.

In short, I believe that programs that bring people together and enrich each other's lives through the creative arts are a key to better Alzheimer's care. Today, art historians, artists, museum professionals, doctors, and scientists across the globe are working with Alzheimer patients. They are discovering that the arts stimulate mental association, sociability, and physical healing.

I am also convinced that many people are waiting to mobilize arts programs and become positive, engaged forces in improving the lives of afflicted persons. And I am pleased to say that the following chapters will provide both inspiration and information to them as they meet the challenges of Alzheimer's disease. With the help of this book, we can expand the power of the arts to open new connections between afflicted persons and their worlds.

Dr. Robert Butler, who died in July 2010, was a pioneering researcher on aging and geriatric medicine and Alzheimer's disease. The author of over 300 books and articles, he was a tireless advocate for engaged activity throughout the later years of life. He was the founding Director of the National Institute on Aging at the National Institutes of Health, the Alzheimer's Association, and the International Longevity Center in New York.

2 Creativity and Art in Promoting Health and Coping with Alzheimer's

Gene D. Cohen, M.D., Ph.D.

We are at the second major turning point in the contemporary focus on aging; that of looking beyond problems to potential.

Promoting Health in Later Life: *The Creativity and Aging Study*

Does creatively engaging older adults in artistic activity offer any hope of improving their general and mental health and social activities? The answer appears to be "yes!" and it offers hope to many who seek to ameliorate the effects of Alzheimer's disease and other memory disorders on their family members or patients.

The *Creativity and Aging Study* is the informal name of a multi-site national research project, *The Impact of Professionally Conducted Cultural Programs on the Physical Health, Mental Health, and Social Functioning of Older Adults.*[1] The study was conducted to explore how creative engagement on the part of older adults relates to their health. What was learned was that efforts at health promotion and prevention among older adults can only go so far when restricted to targeting problems. Ultimately, promoting

---

1 Cohen M.D., Ph.D., Gene et al., *The Impact of Professionally Conducted Cultural Programs on Older Adults*, http://www.nea.gov/resources/accessibility/CnA-Rep4-30-06.pdf April 2006.

health with aging is perhaps best realized when potential is tapped through creative engagement while problems are also addressed.

The *Creativity and Aging Study* was the first formal study, using an experimental or quasi-experimental design involving a comparison group, examining the influence of professionally-conducted, participatory art programs on the general health, mental health and social functioning of older persons. It was designed to draw upon the underlying mechanisms that have been shown to influence positive health outcomes in older persons. Results reveal significant positive differences in the intervention group (those involved in intensive participatory art programs) as compared to a group not involved in intensive cultural programs. I was the primary investigator for the study, which was coordinated by the Center on Aging, Health & Humanities at The George Washington University.

The study began in 2001 with a grant from the National Endowment for the Arts, in coordination with five other federal and non-federal sponsors, including the National Institutes of Health and the National Retired Teachers Association/AARP. The grant was for the purpose of conducting a rigorous national study examining the effects of community-based art programs on the health and functioning of older adults. The study compared the physical and mental health and social functioning of 150 older persons involved in the arts programs (the intervention group) to a similar group of 150 adults not in such programs (the control group). All the participants were age 65 or older and most were living independently when the study started. Both groups were similar in their health and functioning at the start of the study. The adults who were not in the arts group were free to socialize, attend classes, or do any of their normal activities, including art, although none in the control group became involved in rigorous and sustained participatory art programs. *The aim was to see if it was the* **creativity** *involved in the arts programs that made a difference, rather than the mere fact that these participants were engaged in a regular, structured social situation.*

The arts groups met for 35 weekly meetings—analogous to a college course. There were also between-session assignments, as well as exhibitions and concerts. For example, a chorale at one site gave some ten concerts a year in addition to their regular weekly practice sessions.

Each person's health and social functioning were assessed with comprehensive questionnaires at the beginning of the programs, at the half-way mark and again at the end—two years after starting. The hypothesis was that the intervention group, who participated in the arts programs, would show *less decline* than the control group, who did not participate in those programs. In fact, the initial results exceeded these expectations. Many people in the arts groups *stabilized* their health—not declining at all. And some actually *improved* their health. These results occurred in a group of people with an average age of 80—which is greater than the current life expectancy!

Here are the major findings from the first phase of the study.[2] Compared to the control group, those who participated in the community arts program:

- Had better health after one year. Those in the control group reported that their health was not as good after the same elapsed time.

- Had fewer doctor visits, although both groups had more visits compared to a year earlier.

- Used fewer medications, although, again, both groups increased their medication usage.

- Felt less depressed.

- Were less lonely.

- Had higher morale.

---

2   The first phase was conducted in the Washington, D.C. area, where the singing groups were directed by Jeanne Kelly from the Levine School of Music. Similar paired study groups were researched in Brooklyn at the "Elders Shar the Arts, under the direction of Susan Perlstein, and in San Francisco at the Center for Elders and Youth in the Arts, under the direction of Jeff Chapline. Data still under analysis at these two sites reflect results moving in the same direction as the Washington, D.C. findings.

- Were more socially active and more active than at the start of the study. Those in the control group were less socially active compared to a year earlier.

All results were statistically significant, reflecting real differences between the intervention group and the control group.

In summary: better health and improved social activity for the intervention group; not as good health and less social activity for the control group.

Historical Context for the Study

We are at the second major turning point in the contemporary focus on aging: that of looking beyond problems to potential. The focus on problems of the aging reflected the first major turning point, through the launching of the field of Geriatrics. The new focus on potential has profound possibilities for advancing health maintenance and health promotion efforts. Societal interest in later life potential is soaring, and it is in this context that a project studying how cultural programs affect older persons could not be more timely.

Theoretical Background for the Study

The theoretical background for this study built upon several major bodies of gerontologic research addressing underlying mechanisms that promote health with aging, especially those of (1) sense of control, and (2) social engagement. Studies on aging show that when older persons experience a sense of control—e.g., a sense of mastery in what they are doing—positive health outcomes are observed.[3] Similarly, when older individuals are in situations with meaningful social engagement with others, positive health outcomes are also observed.[4]

---

3   Rodin, J. Aging and health: Effects of the sense of control. Science. (1986) 233(4770): 1271-1276 and Rodin, J. Sense of control: Potentials for intervention. Annals of the American Academy of Policy and Social Science (1989) 503: 29-42.

4   Avlund, K., M. T. Damsgaard, and B. E. Holstein. Social relations and mortality: An eleven year follow-up study of 70-year-old men and women in Denmark. Social Science and Medicine (1998) 47(5): 635-643. and Bennett, K. M. Low level social

Biological studies reveal the involvement of mind-immune system pathways playing a protective role, as described in research on psychoneuroimmunology.[5] In this study, both of these dimensions—individual sense of control and social engagement—were combined. Each time a study participant attended an art class, for example, he or she experienced a renewed sense of control—of ongoing individual mastery. Since all of the art programs involved participation and interpersonal interaction with others, social engagement was high.

In all three study sites, there were numerous qualitative reports of participating individuals in the arts programs describing a sense of satisfaction and exhilaration because their performance exceeded their expectations and actually improved. Their growing sense of control was readily apparent. The artists involved with the various groups reported how the repeated success of the various participants profoundly affected their motivation and desire to continue. They consistently reported high self-esteem and mood as the involvement continued. This was well-reflected by a 94-year-old woman in the Washington, D. C., chorale, who shared the following:

> *I'm 94 years old and wasn't sure I could sing, and was even less sure that I could follow the notes. [Becoming increasingly animated] But I found that I could sing! In fact, I'm improving! And, I can't believe it, but I'm finding it easier*

engagement as a precursor of mortality among people in later life. Age and Ageing (2002) 31(3): 165-168. and Glass. T. A., C, M. de Leon. B.A. Marottoli. and L. F. Berkman. Population based study of social and productive activities as predictors of survival among elderly Americans. British Medical Journal (1999) 3 19: 478-483.

5   Pert, C. B., Dreher, H. E., &Ruff, M. R.(1998). The psychosomatic network: Foundations of mind-body medicine. Alternative Therapy and Health Medicine, 4(4), 30-41. and Kiecolt-Glaser, J. K., L. McGuire, T. F. Robles. and R. Glaser. Emotions, morbidity, and mortality: New perspectives from psychoneuroimmunology Annual Renew of Psychology (2002) 53: 83-107. and Lutgendorf, S. K. and L S. Costanzo. Psychoneuroimmunology and health psychology: An integrative model. Brain, Behavior. and Immunity (2003) 17(4): 225-232. and Lutgendorf, S. K., R P. Vitaliano, I Tripp-Reimcr. J. H. Harvey and D. M. Lubaroff. Sense of coherence moderates the relationship between life stress and natural killer cell activity in healthy older adults. Psychology and Aging (1999) 14(4): 552-563.

*and easier to read the notes! I am so glad I decided to take
a chance and join the chorale. This has been one of the most
important experiences of my life. I hope it will never stop. My
daughter feels the same way about it.*

The significance of the art programs per se is that they foster
sustained involvement because of their beauty and productivity.
They keep the participants involved week after week, compounding
positive effects being achieved. Many general activities and physical
exercises do not have this highly engaging, thereby sustaining,
quality.

Conclusions from The Creativity and Aging Study

These remarkable results have attracted attention in both scientific
and lay circles. Clearly, the community-based art programs had
a real effect on health promotion and disease prevention. These,
in turn, supported the independence of the individuals and their
ability to live in their communities and appeared to be reducing
risk factors driving the need for long term care.

The Positive Impact of Creativity on Illness with Aging

Art as Therapy for Illness Among Older Persons

There is a long history of case reports and observational studies
on the impact of art and art therapy on alleviating or coping
with illness in later life. A classic illustration is the experience of
Elizabeth Layton. Until her late sixties, she had experienced a long
chronic history of debilitating depression, going back to her young
adulthood. She had received considerable medical and psychiatric
treatment, but still her depression was unremitting. Then, at age 68,
she enrolled in an art course, examined herself in her looking glass
and wondered if she could draw a self-portrait. To her surprise
and elation, she was able to draw with excellence. This launched a
20-year painting career and associated fame. Her self-applied art
therapy put her depression in complete remission.

    We may even find illuminating parallels in literature. The
role of creative interventions in altering the course of illness is

dramatically captured in the case history of Ebenezer Scrooge.[6] Suffering from an undiagnosed chronic depression, the aging Scrooge was the beneficiary of help from an interdisciplinary outreach team making a home visit to Scrooge in 1843—more than 100 years before the community outreach programs of the 20th Century. The team of three art therapists took advantage of Scrooge's increased late life developmental capacity for conflict resolution. They applied psychodynamic dream work and creative guided imaging techniques, more than 50 years before Freud's classic work *The Interpretation of Dreams*. The outcome was a breakthrough that enabled Scrooge to be released from his depression and to utilize his freed-up energy to help the Cratchit family and Tiny Tim. *A Christmas Carol* is a classic portrayal of the role of creative engagement, allowing us to cope with adversity, find a new way of dealing with the world, and get out of a rut, regardless of age.

Creativity and Alzheimer's Disease

The role for creating opportunities and interventions is now being recognized even in the area of dementing illnesses, which are disorders considered the antithesis of creativity. Willem de Kooning illustrated this well. Despite being afflicted with Alzheimer's disease, de Kooning demonstrated the important phenomenon of possessing an area of preserved skill. All of us have certain skills or interests that we have more highly developed than others—usually an area where we have, in some manner, been creatively engaged. The challenge is to help affected individuals find those areas and have an opportunity to tap them. The result is a quality of life that is increased by the satisfaction of being able to use that residual capacity. Though diagnosed and impaired with Alzheimer's disease, de Kooning still retained some reserve creative capacity to paint, allowing him to continue to produce work sought after by museums. He did so for a few years and then continued painting for several years beyond that, nearly up to the time he died.

---

6   Reported in A Christmas Carol; Dickens, C; 1843

Memory vs. Imagination

Perhaps the ultimate illustration of the universal capacity and resiliency of creative expression can be seen with Alzheimer's disease, where when memory fails in a major way, the creative process of imagination can still be mobilized. The satisfaction of being able to access one's imagination, even when limited, compensates in part for the frustration associated with failing memory. Anne Basting's research with her *TimeSlips Creative Storytelling Project* poignantly demonstrates the persistence of imagination triggered by evocative narrative in the face of failing memory.[7]

The following is a dialogue that illustrates the presence and creative role of imagination in dementia when coping with memory loss. It takes place between the author and his mother shortly after she had a series of small strokes that decimated her memory. The conversation takes place the day after her 90th birthday, which had been a wonderful and very successful family event. The author's mother had had a great time.

> Son: *How was your 90th birthday party?*
> Mother: *I'm sorry; I have no recall of it. But I heard I had a good time.*
> (*The son switches the structure of the conversation from memory mode to imagination mode.*)
> Son: *What would having a good time at your birthday be like?*
> Mother: *Having a lot of family there.*
> Son: *You did have a lot of family there. Would you have a birthday cake?*
> Mother: *Sure.*
> Son: *Would the cake have 90 candles?*
> Mother: *I hope not.*

---

7   See www.timesplips.org. The TimeSlips creative storytelling method opens storytelling to everyone by replacing the pressure to remember with encouragement to imagine.

Not being able to recall the party had given my mother distress. Being able to respond to imagination-prompting questions gave her a sense of satisfaction to be creatively engaged.

Problems vs. Potential:
Signs and Symptoms vs. Strengths and Satisfactions

Even if one applies state-of-the-art medical treatment optimally for Alzheimer's disease patients, their quality of life is still severely impaired, especially by the time that they reach the moderately severe to severe stages of the disorder. Medical treatments focus on signs and symptoms that interfere with functioning and cause discomfort. These clinical problems include memory impairment, depression, agitation and psychosis. Treatments here help with suffering and coping, but quality of life remains very compromised.

What else can one do? From my 35 years of clinical work and research with individuals suffering with major memory disorders, I have learned that beyond *signs* and *symptoms*, two other "S" concepts have intervention significance: residual areas of *strengths* (or skills) and *satisfactions*. These areas of strengths and satisfactions do not reflect clinical problems, but rather individual potential, even in the face of decline. We all have them to varying degrees. Tapping into these residual areas of strengths and satisfactions enhances quality of life for both the patient and the family. The process responds to the person as a person. The examples of Willem de Kooning and Hilda Gorenstein (Hilgos), the subject of other chapters in this book, are illustrations of this point.

Interventions that Enhance the Quality of Life

Too often one hears the unqualified statement that "there is no treatment for Alzheimer's disease." This reflects either a misunderstanding or a misrepresentation of intervention opportunities for this and related disorders. What more accurately characterizes clinical reality is that there is no treatment that can prevent, cure, reverse or arrest the progression of Alzheimer's disease. But, as with other chronic and progressive disorders, there is a range of clinical and psychosocial interventions that can alleviate symptoms and suffering and maximize coping at different points in time or stages during the course of the disorder. There are interventions that can improve the quality of life for both those who suffer from Alzheimer's disease and their families.

I will describe two such quality of life-enhancing products that I have developed and that were awarded First Place in the Blair L. Sadler International Healing Arts Competition, administered by the Society for the Arts in Health Care. The first, a project involving video biographies, was funded by The Helen Bader Foundation. The second, the development of the first board game for Alzheimer's disease and related disorders, was supported by the National Institute on Aging. Both projects employ the same concept, but with different media. The video biographies use images. The board game uses biographical flash cards that have images similar to or the same as those in the video biographies. These products are designed for patients and families struggling with dementia.

Shared Goals of the Video Biographies and the Board Game

The video biographies and the board game share the following goals.

- To alter in a positive way the experience of a devastating illness through providing quality of life-increasing intervals of time. The interventions don't alter the progression, but they improve the experience of shared time.

- To provide valued one-on-one opportunities with the patient to structure meaningful time. Especially in the nursing home, one-on-one time is hard to come by except for purposes of feeding and hygiene.

- To attract visitors who often feel uncomfortable visiting individuals with dementia. The structure provided by the video and its commentary and by the game with its informative flash cards greatly reduces visitor anxiety about what communication can and will take place.

- To foster an intergenerational process, since young family members or young volunteers are often involved in producing the individualized videos and games.

- To improve staff perception of the patient as a person, thereby improving the care of the person.

The Video Biographies (TR-Bios)

The video biographies are known as Therapeutic/Restorative Biographies, or TR-Bios for short, because they help restore meaningful relationships with significant others and bring back, if only briefly, wonderful memories. Families themselves can make the TR-Bios or volunteers can work with families to create them. Often college or graduate students who like working with media are terrific here, adding a warm intergenerational component to the process.

Families are instructed to obtain stories that reflect happy or interesting events for the Alzheimer patient over the course of his or her life. These stories are synthesized and portrayed similarly to the way Ken Burns portrayed the history of the Civil War and the story of baseball on his Public Broadcasting System television series Family photo snapshots are videotaped (and thereby enlarged on the TV screen) and accompanied by commentary. The commentary allows even a new volunteer with no knowledge of the patient to share meaningful time and point out personal details to the patient as informed by the commentary.

If there were favorite stories of the patient, these can be presented by someone who tells them well. If there are associations that might enhance the memory of an event, these too can be incorporated—whether in the form of images, commentary, or even music. Interviews with significant others can also be videotaped and incorporated in the TR-Bios.

Basically, TR-Bio content is sought to attract patient interest and pleasure to the maximum extent possible, and then presented in the most personally engaging visual and auditory manner. A non-pressure *commentary* form of conversation, as opposed to a conventional, but often frustrating, *question-and-answer* format is typically recommended.

The Board Game

The recently-produced, patented board game, *Making Memories Together*,™ is a noncompetitive game where everybody is on the same team, collaborating as necessary on moves.[8] The game consists of a colorful playing board with four different categories of squares: People, Animals, Favorite Things, and Special Places & Events. Players roll a special die with actual numbers on it rather than the traditional dots, moving to one of the squares on the board. Because everybody is on the same team, there is only one marker, further reducing the likelihood of confusion. If you land on the "People Square," for example, there is a pile of "Memory Cards" of different members of the family that have been individually prepared, with pictures on one side and text on the other, all designed to promote quality shared time. The memory cards are then discussed and the game continues as other squares are landed upon and their corresponding memory cards discussed.

The *Making Memories Together* board

The research on both the TR-Bios and the board game revealed significantly superior results when compared to a visit as usual

---

8   More information about Making Memories Together can be obtained on the web at: http://www.genco-games.com/making-memories.html.

with the family and to control conditions. Patient interest and engagement were greatly enhanced as was satisfaction of the visitors. Another poignant feature of both the TR-Bios and the board game is that when the person with the dementia dies, the TR-Bios and board game in effect become exit gifts, leaving the family with wonderful family biographies that they otherwise might never have had, facilitated by their loved one who could no longer tell his or her own story. They contribute to a continuing presence described by the Scottish poet Thomas Campbell: "To live in the hearts we leave behind is not to die."

Dr. Gene Cohen, who died in November 2009, was one of the early leaders in geriatric research and served as the Acting Director of the National Institute on Aging. He was the founding Director of the Center on Aging, Health and Humanities at The George Washington University, where he was also Professor of Psychiatry and Professor of Health Care Sciences. He was also the founding editor of the American Journal of Geriatric Psychiatry.

3 Art and the Brain

Avertano Noronha, M.B.B.S., M.D.

...creative activity...engages the 'I' in us,
giving us a sense of accomplishment.

While creativity can express itself in virtually any domain, art may well illustrate how the brain processes creative endeavors when affected by disease. The remarkable improvement in well-being in the artist Hilgos following a return to painting is the impetus for an enquiry into the effect of neurological degenerative diseases on artistic expression and strategies to encourage artistic activity in individuals with cognitive impairment.

Neurological Diseases That Affect Cognitive Function

I would like to provide the lay reader a brief description of the neurological diseases that affect cognitive function. Dementia is a term that has been used to describe a decline in memory and intellectual abilities that interferes with activities of daily life. It is important to note that the diseases that will be discussed, Alzheimer's disease and Frontotemporal dementia, cause a progressive decline in intellectual function. As we age, it is not uncommon to experience occasional forgetfulness. This need not be a cause for alarm as it can occur without any evidence of disease. If there is a concern, a neurologist would be able to address the significance of the memory disorder. Metabolic conditions such as nutritional deficiencies can be diagnosed with blood tests and are easily treated. Dr. Lawrence Lazarus's comments in Chapter 4 provide a good overview of the importance of a careful psycho-medical-social evaluation.

Minimal Cognitive Dysfunction (MCD) is a term used to describe a mild impairment in memory testing. Follow-up testing is recommended; not all patients with MCD go on to develop Alzheimer's disease.

Alzheimer's disease (AD) is a progressive and fatal neurological disease. It is the most common form of dementia worldwide; approximately 5 million Americans are living with AD.

Cognitive impairment occurs in other neurological diseases, such as *vascular dementia* secondary to strokes, and in degenerative neurological diseases such as *Frontotemporal dementia* (FTD), *Parkinson's disease* and *Lewy body disease*. Hallucinations are an early feature of Lewy body disease and can occur in AD.[1] Strokes in the posterior part of the brain, the occipital area which subserves vision, can have an effect on the appreciation and performance of art.

Comparing Alzheimer's Disease to Frontotemporal Disease

The clinical and pathological features are distinctive for each of the degenerative neurological diseases. I have chosen to describe the two major progressive neurological diseases with cognitive decline, and I will compare and contrast AD and FTD.

In Alzheimer's disease, the distinctive pathological features are formation of amyloid[2] plaques and neurofibrillary[3] tangles. Beta-amyloid peptides[4] are deposited in the brain and form plaques. Disruption of neurofilaments (Tau protein) in neurons and their processes forms neurofibrillary tangles in AD.

---

1   Dysken, MW, P Fovall, CM Harris, JM Davis, and A Noronha. 1982. "Lecithin administration in Alzheimer dementia." *Neurology* 32:1203.

2   Amyloid is a hard, waxy deposit consisting of protein and polysaccharides that results from the degeneration of tissue.

3   Neurofibrils are long, thin, microscopic fibrils that run through the body of a neuron.

4   Peptides are compounds containing two or more amino acids.

The core deficit in Alzheimer's disease is memory loss; older memories are relatively preserved early in the illness and other systems are functional. Eventually, progressive degeneration occurs in several brain systems resulting in behavioral and psychiatric symptoms. Understanding the pathology of AD has resulted in the development of medications that initially provide improvement of memory and behavioral symptoms; eventually, the disease progresses. Therapies that could prevent the deposition of amyloid protein in the brain are in clinical trials; if effective, it would be important to diagnose and treat AD in the earliest stages.

Frontotemporal dementia can be mistaken for AD. In frontotemporal dementia, mutations in the normal Tau protein cause degeneration of the neurons. FTD is a progressive neurological disease that affects the frontal lobes and is a consequence of disruption of neurofilaments that transport nutrients in neural processes. The clinical features of FTD are due to a lack of inhibition in brain areas and range from changes in personality to impairment in planning and social functioning. Individuals with FTD may make unwise decisions about finances or personal matters. The frontal and temporal lobes are affected; symptoms of disinhibition are consequent to disease in the frontal lobes of the brain. Difficulties with language characterize one of the forms of FTD known as primary progressive aphasia.

The Effect of AD and FTD on Art and Music

I will now discuss art and music in AD and FTD and examine the effects of each disease on art and music.

Visual art is one expression of neurological function that is mediated predominantly by the right hemisphere of the brain; in contrast, the left hemisphere has inhibitory effects on artistic expression. Inhibitory and excitatory mechanisms interact in harmony. Brain diseases such as dementia could change this harmony and alter artistic expression. The paintings of William Utermohlen and Willem de Kooning, both of whom had Alzheimer's disease, changed dramatically after the onset of their illnesses.

William Utermohlen's self-portraits done during the course of Alzheimer's disease show a progressive decrease in detail and perspective. Loss of visual-spatial abilities occur in AD, and Utermohlen's paintings showed a decline in form and perspective. His self-portraits show a progressive change in definition that may be described as indistinct. He was aware of his errors but said that he was unable to correct them.

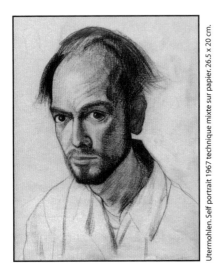 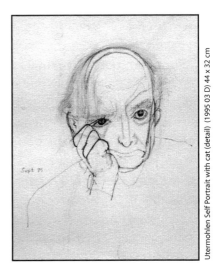

William Utermohlen's self-portraits, created in 1967 and 1995, show a progressive decrease in detail and perspective.

Willem de Kooning, a leader in the abstract expressionist art movement, was known for his vibrant slashes of color and shifting foregrounds and backgrounds. After he developed Alzheimer's in the 1980's, the lines in his paintings continued to allude to the biomorphic shapes of his earlier works, but had less detail, becoming cleaner and more sparse.

The effect of disinhibition can sometimes be seen in the art of patients with FTD, causing their art to be vivid. Interestingly, some individuals with FTD, including the primary progressive aphasia type, can develop an interest in art, an interest which may not have been present prior to the illness.

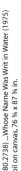
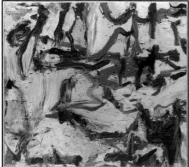
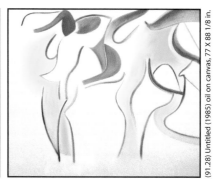

Willem de Kooning's 1975 painting (left) still shows complexity of detail. By 1985 (right) his lines had become cleaner and more sparse.

With regard to music, one form of memory for music can be preserved in patients with Alzheimer's disease. Implicit or procedural memory for music—the ability to play a musical instrument—may be spared in musicians with AD. In contrast, explicit musical memory, which is the recognition of familiar or unfamiliar melodies, is often impaired.

Many of us are familiar with *Bolero*, composed by Ravel in 1928 when he was 53 years old. The score alternates between two melodic themes, repeating the pair eight times over 340 bars with increasing volume and layer of instruments. The score holds to two simple, alternating staccato base lines. Ravel eventually developed cognitive difficulties, as revealed by errors in his musical scores and in his personal letters. The nature of Ravel's so called "mystery illness" was unknown at that time. The elements of repetition in the Bolero score have drawn the attention of neuroscientists to the possibility that Ravel's later illness was FTD.[5]

The Effect of Creative Activities on AD and FTD

The story of the artist, Hilgos, who suffered from Alzheimer's disease, is a compelling example of the well-being that resulted from a return to her creative activity, painting, which was, for her,

---

5   See William W. Seeley *et al*, "Unravelling Bolero: progressive aphasia, transmodal creativity and the right posterior neocortex," Brain Journal (2008), v131, pp 39-49, Francois Sellal, "Letter to the Editor," Brain Journal (2008), v131, e98, and William W. Seeley *et al*, "Letter to the Editor," Brain Journal (2008), v131, e99.

the mainspring of her life. I have had the privilege of observing the paintings and sculptures of this artist. The paintings subsequent to the illness show no decline in composition and no change to an abstract form; the form of the objects is maintained, but is simplified.

One may ask whether activity in the creative arts could induce well-being in other individuals with dementia who are not accomplished artists such as Hilgos. *In my opinion, it is the creative activity that stimulates the brain in a manner distinct from other physical and group activities; it engages the "I" in us, giving us a sense of accomplishment.*

Preliminary studies of the effect of artistic activity and exposure to art in patients with cognitive decline show that creative activity reduces depression and isolation. A study of patients in the early and middle stages of Alzheimer's disease who participated in an art therapy program showed that the individuals demonstrated significantly more interest, sustained attention, pleasure, self-esteem and normalcy during participation in the art therapy program than individuals who participated in more traditional adult day center activities, such as current events and crafts.

Meet Me at MoMA is a program for early and moderate AD; museum educators at the Museum of Modern Art escort patients and relatives to selected art works for observation and discussion. Trained observers who have worked with patients with AD reported that patients and their caregivers were very involved in observing the paintings and in discussing the art. The well spouse was able to see that the ill spouse could take part in ordinary activity. The program provided intellectual stimulation and social interaction. It engaged the "I" and provided enrichment that is conducive to neurogenesis (birth of new neurons). As word spread in the AD community, MoMA was contacted by 40 other museums and has now started the *MoMA Alzheimer's Project.*[6]

These observational studies will need to be confirmed by modern imaging techniques (functional MRI) that record brain

---

6   For more information, see http://www.moma.org/meetme/.

activity in different regions of the brain before and after a well-designed course of art therapy.

The Effect of Physical Exercise and Enriched Environments on AD

One may question if there is a biological basis for a response to physical exercise or enriched environments in Alzheimer's disease. It has long been held that the adult brain does not have the capacity to make new neurons. This notion has recently changed. It is now well-accepted that proliferation of neural stem/precursor cells (NSCs) occurs in the adult brain, primarily, in the dentate gyrus of the hippocampus. The hippocampus is a structure in the temporal lobe that is important in memory function; surgical removal of this structure in both hemispheres results in the inability to consolidate memories. The affected individual is always living in the past.[7] Hippocampal neurons degenerate in AD. It has been suggested that neurogenesis in the normal adult central nervous system plays a role in learning and memory, adaptation to novel environments, and in recovery from injury or disease. Proliferation of neural stem/precursor cells declines dramatically before middle age.

Physical exercise has been recommended to individuals with AD. Marcus Tullius Cicero stated, circa 65 BC, "It is exercise alone that supports the spirits, and keeps the mind in vigor."[8] John Adams, the second president of the United States, said, "Exercise invigorates, and enlivens all the faculties of body and of mind... It spreads a gladness and satisfaction over our minds and qualifies us for every sort of business, and every sort of pleasure."[9]

Physical exercise is known to promote adult neurogenesis in mice. Mandatory treadmill running for five weeks was shown

---

7   Dr. Brenda Milner, a pioneer in the study of memory, was the first to study the effects of damage to the medial temporal lobe on memory. She described these in the most famous patient in cognitive neuroscience, Henry Gustav Molaison, known as HM.

8   Cicero, Marcus Tullius. *M. T. Cicero's Cato Major, Or Discourse On Old Age: Addressed to Titus Pomponius Atticus*. With explanatory notes by Benj. Franklin, LL. D. London: Fielding and Walker, 1778, p.77.

9   De Mooy, Kees. *The Wisdom of John Adams*. New York: Citadel, 2003, p. 46.

to increase hippocampal neurogenesis and improve learning in experimental animals.

There is, in addition, a significant effect of enrichment (exposure to novel stimuli) on neurogenesis. Transgenic mice that carry the pre-senilin gene mutations for familial Alzheimer's disease were exposed to an enriched environment in a laboratory. They were kept in large cages which allowed them to explore running wheels, colored tunnels, toys, and chewable objects. They spent three hours each day for a month exposed to these opportunities. Neurogenesis developed in the dentate gyrus of the hippocampus in these animals. The above experiments validate the usefulness of exercise and exposure to novel stimuli in normal aging and in Alzheimer's disease.

Evidence for humans is beginning to be published. Exercise improved cognitive function in patients with AD who were randomized in a clinical trial to either of two groups: a treatment group that engaged in an exercise program over a period of 6 months or a control group that did not exercise but received educational literature. Cognitive scores (ADAS-Cog) were significantly better in the group that exercised when assessed 18 months later.[10]

To conclude, Hilgos said it succinctly: "I remember better when I paint." In expressing this personal insight, Hilgos opened a door to exploring unsuspected potential in many persons afflicted with memory loss.

Avertano Noronha, M.B.B.S., M.D., is Associate Professor in the Department of Neurology, the Committee on Immunology and the College at the University of Chicago. His major area of interest is in multiple sclerosis; additional fields of interest include lupus and the vasculitides, Huntington's disease, Alzheimer's disease and the neurological complications of pregnancy.

---

10 Lautenschlager, NT et al. JAMA 2008; 300: 1028-1037.

4 Restoring the Sense of Self: Hilgos's Story

Lawrence W. Lazarus, M.D., D.L.F.A.P.A.

> *Dormant skills and abilities can be reactivated, not only to restore self-esteem, but to improve overall functioning and mood.*

Interacting with the Alzheimer's Patient

Alzheimer's disease, the most common cause of memory impairment in the elderly, and other memory disorders have a profound, devastating effect not only on the person suffering from the illness but also on the family. It is a terrifying experience to realize that one's cognitive and intellectual functioning, the very essence of one's sense of self and self-esteem, is gradually being eroded. All the interpersonal, social, occupational, and intellectual skills gradually acquired and refined over a lifetime of experience undergo a gradual, painstaking deterioration.

Coping with Alzheimer's Disease

In an attempt to cope with a decline in memory, the afflicted person may deny the impairment, use humor to minimize it, and become annoyed at others who try to correct cognitive errors. There is an exaggeration of life-long defense mechanisms such as denial, rationalization, intellectualization, and sometimes projection (e.g., accusations that someone has stolen misplaced items). Memory for recent events is usually more impaired than longer-term memory. For example, a person may not remember where the keys or wallet were placed, but can remember significant names and experiences from the past. Fortunately, special skills and attributes developed earlier in life, such as artistic and musical abilities, may be preserved. This relative preservation of significant memories and skills acquired earlier in life provides family and health professionals a window of opportunity for working therapeutically with the afflicted person.

The Value of Creative Activities

Dr. Robert Butler, the first Director of the U.S. National Institute on Aging, and Dr. Gene Cohen, Professor of Psychiatry at George Washington University, have written extensively about the therapeutic value of encouraging and fostering memory-impaired persons to re-engage in previously developed artistic and other creative activities. Reminiscing about positive events and accomplishments enhances self-esteem and a positive sense of self. Dr. Cohen has advocated that families of demented persons who are living in nursing homes or assisted living facilities bring memorabilia and symbols of past accomplishments to remind the afflicted family member of his/her past accomplishments. The memorabilia might include photographs of family members, and the symbols might include trophies and other awards. This also enhances the nursing home staffs' understanding and appreciation of who the afflicted person really was before the illness took its toll.

Educating the Nursing Staff

Because it's difficult for the Alzheimer's-afflicted patient to convey to the long term care facility's staff aspects of his/her life such as personality characteristics, past interests, and creative abilities, it's difficult for staff to empathize with and truly know the newly-admitted nursing home resident. The family of the afflicted resident can inform and educate staff about the real nature, essence and personality of their family member to enable staff to empathize with and understand both the verbal and non-verbal behavior of their family member. Showing old photographs or home videos to staff members helps to personalize the true nature of the newly-admitted but "unknown" resident. Some gerontologists have even suggested that the family bring to the nursing home a videotaped interview of their family member during an early stage of the dementia, including commentary from other family members that emphasizes the interests, personality, and accomplishments of the person. This helps staff understand better the behavior and verbalizations of the patient. For example, in Hilda's case, she exclaimed to the art students helping her, "Quick, quick," while holding her right arm outstretched, signaling her desire to paint.

Re-Establishing the Sense of Self

The loving concern shown by Berna Huebner, Hilda's daughter, and other family members toward Hilda demonstrates how dormant skills and abilities can be reactivated, not only to restore self-esteem, but to improve overall functioning and mood. Hilda had been an accomplished artist, traveler, and adventurer. The slow progression of dementia eventually led to her withdrawal from family and from exercising the skills and creativity that gave her pleasure and identity as an artist. Eventual confinement to a nursing home, where staff lacked awareness of who she really was, only reinforced her feelings of isolation and aloneness. Determined to restore her mother's sense of personhood, Berna arranged for interested students from the School of the Art Institute of Chicago to encourage Hilda to resume her artistic interest. The enthusiasm of the students eventually spread to the nursing personnel, who began to take a lively interest in Hilda's burgeoning artistic output. Once the nursing home staff understood and appreciated the latent talents and skills that were an important aspect of Hilda's real self, they interacted more with her, producing a calming effect on her and facilitating higher levels of functioning.

Using Therapeutic Techniques

The following example shows another way staff can use therapeutic techniques. A destructive, angry nursing home patient expresses the delusional belief that he/she is impatiently awaiting a visit from a long-deceased parent. This delusion may be adaptive, in that it represents a fantasized reunion with an idealized, sorely missed parent in order to combat feelings of depression, isolation, and depletion in a nursing home environment perceived as cold and indifferent. Rather than confronting the demented patient with the reality that his/her parent is deceased, a therapeutic response may be to empathize with how much the anticipated visit must mean to the resident. The staff member can then change the subject or engage the patient in some activity.

The Comprehensive Biopsychosocial Evaluation and Treatment Plan.

The comprehensive medical evaluation of an elderly demented individual is a critically important starting point because an accurate diagnosis and thorough understanding of the total person guides the ensuing treatment. Unfortunately, elderly patients presenting to their busy primary care physicians may not be attended with the same thorough evaluation given to a younger patient presenting with similar symptoms.

An excellent model guiding the comprehensive evaluation was developed decades ago by Drs. George Engel and John Romano[1] at the University of Rochester. They conceived of the biopsychosocial model which emphasizes the investigation of biological (or medical), psychological, and social components of the patient's often complex problems. A cultural and religious component is an important addition to this model.

Taking a Detailed History

Undoubtedly, the most important component of the evaluation is a careful, detailed history of the development of the memory and

---

1   The biopsychosocial model is a general model or approach that proposes that biological, psychological (which entails thoughts, emotions, and behaviors), and social factors, all play a significant role in human functioning in the context of disease or illness. Indeed, health is best understood in terms of a combination of biological, psychological, and social factors rather than purely in biological terms. This is in contrast to the traditional, reductionist biomedical model of medicine that suggests every disease process can be explained in terms of an underlying deviation from normal function such as a pathogen, genetic or developmental abnormality, or injury.

associated problems. Typical of Alzheimer's disease, there is a slow progressive impairment of cognitive and intellectual abilities, often accompanied by anxiety or depression. The afflicted person may deny or minimize the problem and become increasingly dependent on spouse or another family member to come up with the word that he/she can't express. Difficulty managing the checkbook and adjusting to even minor changes in routine, along with nighttime wandering or agitation may follow. The afflicted person may misplace belongings and blame the principal care provider, such as the spouse, for stealing from him/her.

Evaluating Medical Problems

Before a tentative diagnosis of Alzheimer's disease can be reached, the physician needs to explore treatable and potentially reversible medical problems that can present as dementia. For example, diseases of the thyroid or other endocrine disorders, vitamin deficiencies such as B12 and folic acid, collagen-vascular diseases such as lupus, anemia, heavy metal poisoning from lead or mercury, head trauma and a whole array of other medical problems may masquerade as a dementing illness. Therefore, extensive blood tests, neurophychological testing and sometimes specialized radiographic scans of the head may need to be performed.

Evaluating Psychological Problems

From a psychological perspective, a profound depression with accompanying apathy, inattention, loss of interest and withdrawal may present as if the patient were demented—a condition sometimes called "pseudodementia." Depression often is a concomitant of a dementia, and aggressive treatment of the former can result in considerable overall improvement. An understanding of the pre-morbid personality of the demented patient can likewise have important treatment applications. There is often an exaggeration of previous personality traits and a regression to more primitive psychological defense mechanisms such as denial and projection (manifested by paranoid accusations) as a way of coping with the frightening realization that one's cognitive and intellectual abilities are deteriorating. Pre-morbid personality traits of passivity or aggressiveness and dependency may become exaggerated. A skilled therapist can encourage and support more adaptive coping mechanisms such as the compulsive use of daily schedules and other memory aids.

Evaluating Sociological Problems

From a sociological standpoint, embarrassment and shame over cognitive impairment may result in avoidance of social interaction. In a like fashion, the spouse, feeling the need to be protective, may avoid informing children and friends about the illness and isolate the spouse and himself/herself from the nurturing companionship of others, resulting in further isolation and withdrawal. The patient may withdraw from the very activities that contributed to a sense of purpose and self-esteem, such as painting, music and former hobbies.

Understanding the Cultural and Religious Background

Understanding the person's and their family's cultural and religious background and beliefs is important in understanding how regular attendance at religious ceremonies can promote socialization and participation in highly valued and remembered activities. It also helps the treatment team understand their attitude toward treatment and possible eventual placement in a long term care facility. For example, persons from certain cultural groups wherein family ties are very strong, such as Hispanic and Asian families, may have a strong preference to care for a family member with advanced dementia at home, even in situations where patient needs become so extensive that placement becomes the only viable alternative.

Using Psychotropic Medications

Oftentimes, intervention by an experienced geriatric psychiatrist or internist utilizing psychiatric medication judiciously along with psychotherapy and family counseling can help stabilize a patient with severe behavioral problems and psychotic symptoms, thus enabling the patient to remain longer in the familiar setting of the family home. The principal caregiver, such as the spouse or son/daughter of the person afflicted with Alzheimer's disease often suffers from emotional exhaustion or depression and can benefit from psychiatric intervention. If the principal caregiver can be helped to become more emotionally stable and to learn effective ways of responding to the afflicted relative, the caregiver can be more proficient and calmer. Caregivers can also benefit from participation in various educational and support groups sponsored by a local chapter of the Alzheimer's Association.

Dr. Lawrence W. Lazarus is currently Assistant Professor of Psychiatry at the University of New Mexico and has a private practice in Santa Fe, New Mexico. He is a Past President of the American Association for Geriatric Psychiatry and a Distinguished Fellow of the American Psychiatric Association. Earlier in his career, he was Director of the Geropsychiatry Fellowship Program and Associate Attending Psychiatrist at Rush Medical College in Chicago and attending psychiatrist to Hilda Gorenstein.

Part II: The Artists' Stories

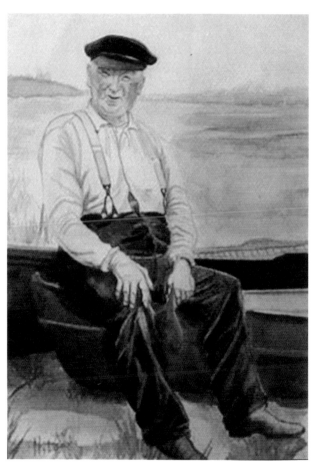

The Lighthouse Keeper by Hilgos, 1962

5 Revelation and Legacy

Berna G. Huebner

> *My mother's unique experience with her*
> *artist student group...is an example of a*
> *new kind of progress and growth people can*
> *have despite aging and memory loss.*

A Brief Portrait of My Mother

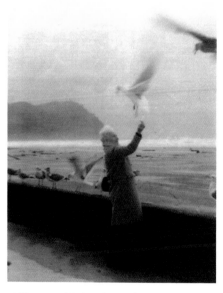

Hilgos with birds at the seaside.

My mother, Hilda Gorenstein, was raised in Portland, Oregon, and started painting in her teens. Around that time, her family moved to Chicago, and after high school my mother continued her studies at the School of the Art Institute of Chicago and graduated in the 1920's. In a profession dominated by men, she chose to call herself Hilgos, a combination of her first and last names and a name that conveyed neither masculine nor feminine identity. She started selling her works to clients in the Chicago area at an early age.

In her twenties, she established herself as a marine painter, painting seascapes, birds, and sailing craft. Soon her work began to make its way into collections not only in the Chicago area but in other parts of the country and the world. When the 1933 Century of Progress World's Fair was being planned in Chicago, the U.S. Navy invited my mother to design and paint 14 enormous murals depicting the history of the Navy. The work remained one of her proudest artistic accomplishments.

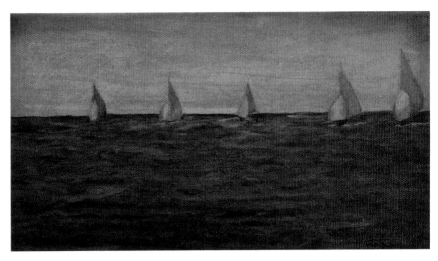

Hilgos painted *Racing Lake Michigan* in 1931.

As the years progressed, my mother's enthusiasm took her into a wide variety of artistic endeavors. She loved experimenting, taking on new challenges, trying new subject matter, new techniques, and new ideas. She was inspired by Asian art and created sculptures and lamps in a Tibetan motif.

My father was proud of my mother's work. He was an attorney professionally and had his own practice. He sometimes worked

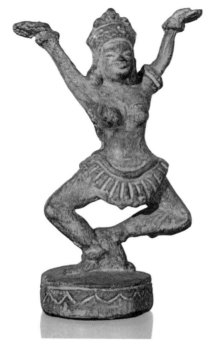

A Tibetan dancer sculpted by Hilgos in 1958

with my mother, creating and carving picture frames for my mother's paintings.

In addition to painting and sculpting, my mother was an avid gardener. Lilac bushes bordered her front yard. Day lilies covered the back. Irises lined the garden outside the sunroom, contrasting with the poppies which bloomed profusely each June. As our dear friend and neighbor, Angie Levenstein, would later say, "Hilda loved her garden. It was entwined with her persona—her eye for color, shapes, harmonies and the movements between. It expressed her appreciation of life and her creative eye. She took pride in her garden, and she shared its beauty and bounty as she did her own accomplishments."

Remembering Mother from childhood, I think of her as tall with beautiful hair. One niece described her as being as graceful as a swan. She always wore very high heels and dressed elegantly. She enjoyed modeling in fashion shows. Mother was positive in spirit, a pillar of strength, appreciative and happy. She was very involved in art, painting and teaching, and was extremely active in the art community, especially at the Art Institute of Chicago.

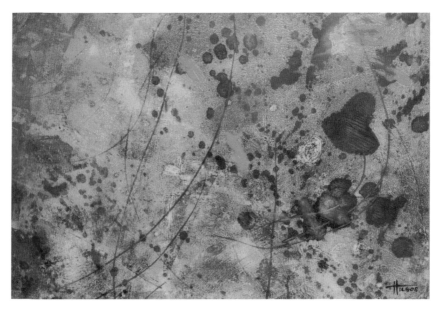

Hilgos created this abstract painting in the 1970s.

Because she spent her childhood on the Oregon coast, she loved birds, especially seagulls, which she frequently painted. She taught my brother and me at a young age to make clay seashells, which she then glued onto a glazed sea green entrance hall wall. She imprinted sea fans on the plaster. Between her art lectures and modeling, she would deliver her newly finished Tibetan sculptures and lamps to the truck entrance of the Merchandise Mart in Chicago. Not yet knowing how to appreciate this kind of endeavor, my brother and I would sit in the back seat of the car and think that everyone's mother had this kind of talent. Sometimes when we would come home from school, she would be giving art lessons to young students, instructing them among other things not to paint the picture in the middle of the page.

I remember waking up in the middle of the night one time to find Mother painting "The Creation," a very colorful picture depicting the earth's beginning. She said she could not sleep; the idea was brimming over in her mind. She felt so inspired.

Although I left home to go to college and later to pursue my own career, I stayed close to my parents. They both continued to work and travel throughout their seventies. In her early eighties, when my mother would become discouraged by the afflictions of age and talk about "closing up shop," my father and I would talk her out of that decision, urging her to find some way to at least keep her hand in her work. I think we knew intuitively—as one of the art students, Robin Barcus-Slonina, later said—that "the creative process is as essential to an artist as breathing, especially after it has been cultivated over the course of a lifetime." Somehow we knew that painting and sculpting were the keys to my mother's vitality.

Even when my husband's and my work took us and our two sons to Paris, I still stayed in close touch with both my parents. I would send my mother postcards and pictures and ask her to create watercolor reproductions of them. Whenever I visited, I would bring all kinds of requests for work.

Confronting Alzheimer's with Art

Both of my parents remained healthy up until their eighties, but, unfortunately, my mother began to develop Alzheimer's then. The care that she needed eventually proved too much for my father. Despite my deep reservations, it was decided in 1995, when she was 91, that my mother should be moved to a nursing home near my brother's and father's homes.

The move was very upsetting for me and disorienting for my mother, who became much more withdrawn in the new environment. It was heartbreaking to see, but even worse to be told by the nursing home staff that it was "no use" trying to work with my mother and that "her lights were out."

Fortunately, as part of developing a true diagnosis of my mother's condition, the nursing home recommended that she be sent to the Rush-Presbyterian St. Luke's Medical Center for an observation period and medical diagnosis. At Rush-Presbyterian I met Dr. Lawrence Lazarus, a geriatric psychiatrist, who thankfully had an open and creative mind. I told him how I thought that my mother's memory might be aided through painting and artwork. I told him I had asked her if she wanted to paint, and she had replied, "Oh yes! I remember better when I paint."

Dr. Lazarus agreed with me and suggested that art students from the School of the Art Institute of Chicago be asked to paint with her. I jumped at the idea and immediately went to put up signs at the Art Institute's job board. Over time, four art students were hired, and they worked with my mother at the nursing home until almost the end of her life. A new family tree was created: the art students, a geriatric psychiatrist, our family, and me. A new language of understanding was generated through the art we created there. A new type of communication developed between us.

My mother started painting again, although it took a couple of months. The works she created at this period in her life reflected her keen eye for color and space. The themes that ran throughout her entire life's work—the sea, birds, sailing—were reflected in her new work. As one of her art students, Robin Barcus-Slonina, would later write:

> The vestiges of her earlier masterful renderings of these subjects remained evident in this late work, although transformed into a new system of spontaneous personal gestures that bordered on the abstract....The trained eyes of the artists who worked with her found the color choices and placement of compositional elements strikingly accomplished.

We were excited to see that, as my mother painted, new recollections would occur and bands of memory would be stimulated. She was aware of this process. It seemed that some of the boats she painted were now functioning as vessels or containers that could store memory for her to be accessed later. By 1997, we created an art show of my mother's work and the work of the students who had painted and sculpted with her. My mother named the show: she called it "Accessible."

Through working with the art students, painting and creating, my mother was able to reintegrate into our world and reconnect with us, despite living in an altered state and suffering from memory loss. Art had played a special role in her life, and now painting enabled her to continue to create, to "talk" with the art students about her work, and to communicate in a way she would not otherwise have done at this time in her life. It was communication both with words and beyond words.

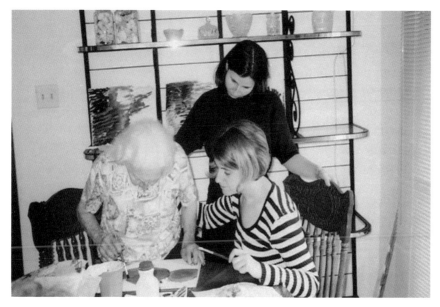

Hilgos painting with art students Robin Barcus-Slonina
(standing) and Jenny Graf Sheppard (seated)

My mother's unique experience with her artist student group was well documented through the artwork itself and is an example of a new kind of progress and growth people can have despite aging and memory loss.

My mother's experience would later be validated by a study entitled "Leisure Activity and the Risk of Dementia in the Elderly,"[1]

---

1   Verghese, J, Lipton, RB, Katz, MJ, et al. "Leisure Activities and the Risk of Dementia in the Elderly." *New England Journal of Medicine.* 2003; 348: 2508-16.

published in June 2003 in the *New England Journal of Medicine*. The authors found that participation in cognitively challenging activities such as chess, dance, cards, and other pursuits, was associated with reduced risk of dementia in the elderly.

Dr. Joseph Coyle, a professor of psychiatry and neuroscience at Harvard Medical School, wrote a commentary on the study entitled "Use It or Lose It—Do Effortful Mental Activities Protect Against Dementia?"[2] He explained how he thought the molecular determinism of Alzheimer's disease could be trumped by something as seemingly simple as a good game of bridge:

> *The effortful mental activity may not only strengthen existing synaptic connections and generate new ones; it may also stimulate neurogenesis especially in the hippocampus. Thus persistent engagement by the elderly in effortful mental activities may promote plastic changes in the brain that circumvent the pathology underlying the symptoms of dementia.*

In addition, Dr. Coyle told a *Washington Post* reporter that "using the mind actually causes rewiring of the brain, sprouting new synapses—it may even cause the generation of new neurons. So psychology trumps biology."[3]

This type of thinking represented a new way of viewing the field of neuroscience. Scientists have started to discover that in many ways the brain is *plastic*, a word that comes from the Greek *plastikos*, which means *malleable*. Thoughts and experiences may actually change neural structure and chemistry.[4]

Unfortunately, this type of understanding of Alzheimer's was not prevalent among the nursing home staff where my mother lived. They saw the progression of my mother's condition as inevitably downward. Their concept of care did not include the idea

---

2   Coyle, J "Use It or Lose It—Do Effortful Mental Activities Protect against Dementia?" *New England Journal of Medicine*. 2003; 348: 2489-2490.

3   Vendantam, Shankar "Mind Games May Trump Alzheimer's: Study Cites Effects of Bridge, Chess." *The Washington Post*. June 19, 2003. p. A01.

4   Ibid.

of helping people to continue to make a contribution to community and family despite current limitations.

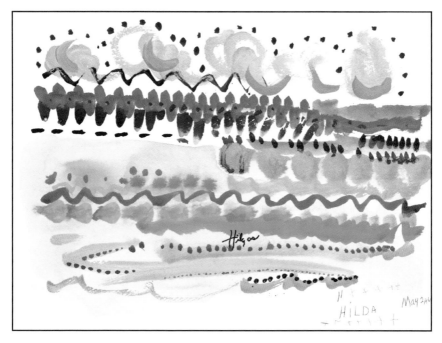

Hilgos created this 1998 painting
while working with the art students.

It became a battle with the staff to allow the art students to paint with my mother. Negotiations took place almost daily to permit the students to enter the nursing facility. "It is too much activity for her," the staff would complain. Sometimes the art students would be seen as troublemakers, as from time to time they would attempt to include other residents in the painting projects. Just when patient interest was piqued, the students would be reprimanded and asked to leave the facility.

Meanwhile, mother was having a wonderful time playing the piano, singing, playing catch, and painting and painting and painting. The art students worked with mother daily for as long as they were allowed. Sometimes when the students were asked to leave, private nurses whom we hired would paint or sing or play catch with her.

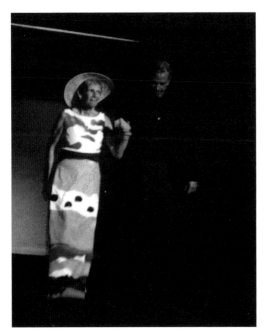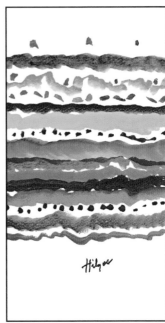

Nancy Paschke models a dress made from fabric printed with Hilgos's artwork and designed by Oscar de la Renta.

When I would arrive at the nursing home, Mother would often say "Here comes the boss, watch out," or "Here comes the real one," revealing the important role that I played and thereby acknowledging that the students had come to play an important role in her life, becoming surrogate children without ever replacing her family and friends. Paintings, art exhibitions, baking, and new faces filled her life.

When my mother died from an unexpected bout of pneumonia at the age of 93, we grieved. But we also celebrated her life. We knew that she had been able to make a contribution right up until the day she died.

My Mother's Legacy: The Hilgos Scholarship Awards

After my mother's death in 1998, our family wanted to continue the work we had begun. And so we established a scholarship in my mother's name, the Hilgos Award. This award provides funding to the School of the Art Institute of Chicago to support and encourage the ongoing process of artistic creation with people who have memory impairment.

To announce the scholarship, we held a gala dinner and fundraiser at the School of the Art Institute. The focal point of the evening was a fashion show, the suggestion of Charles Nolan, the fashion designer for Ellen Tracy, Anne Klein, and his own line of designs. My mother's artwork was screened onto fabrics that were then fashioned into clothing for seniors and handicapped people. Oscar de la Renta, Ellen Tracy, Jean-Charles Castelbajac, and art students designed the outfits. Other prominent participants included Marisa Berenson, who narrated, School Dean Carol Becker, Dr. Larry Lazarus, and Chicago artists Nancy and Ed Pashke.

In his remarks, School President Tony Jones described the Hilgos students as "... pathfinders, whose love and dedication and inquisitive spirit changed Hilgos' life, and by extension the lives of many others…" Such projects, he said, have been "seminal in the creation of a worldwide movement."

The Hilgos Award has since continued in this spirit. As the Chicago Tribune reported: "Across the city senior citizens are getting in touch with their creative sides, and students from the School of the Art Institute of Chicago are helping them do it."

Today four students a year receive the Hilgos Award and continue this truly life-giving work. From their many remarkable stories, I have chosen a few to represent the extraordinary work being done by these inspired young professionals.[5]

One project was a multi-sensory approach to art, designed by Sara Bennett-Steele for the residents at the Lieberman assisted

---

5   Thank you to Katharine Houpt, Sophie Canadé, and Laura Evonne Steinman for their project descriptions, and to Ronna Lazar Heftman for her description of Sara Bennett-Steele's project. Other award winners with descriptions of their highly diversified projects can be found on the Scholarship tab at www.hilgos.org.

living home. As residents and their caregivers walked down their hallways, they would stop to smell, touch, hear, and see a wonderful variety of special stimuli. One sniff of spice or coffee could help a resident relive a special time. Listening to music or a message on a telephone could elicit a thoughtful reaction—or provoke a laugh. Sometimes, just touching the yellow feathers that were mounted on the wall would bring a smile to a resident's face.

Award winner Katharine Houpt developed partnerships between three older adults (two with moderate dementia) at an adult day service and three six-year-old girls at a community center. To build relationships, the participants exchanged artworks with Katharine acting as intermediary, delivering art to the decorated mailboxes each participant created. The exchange became an ongoing conversation with art as the language, as participants in each group created new art in response to the art they received. The art exchange was an enriching avenue for communication, self-expression, and community building for both sets of participants.

Award winner Sophie Canadé believes that the stories of our lives are recorded in and expressed by all parts of our bodies. She has helped to organize Motion Pictures, an art therapy group that capitalizes on the links between motion, emotion, and cognition. She designed the program for older residents of a retirement community, encouraging them to employ both their dominant and non-dominant hands to make large-scale drawings, inviting physical motion in combination with visual expression to recover life experiences that may no longer have been accessible to cognitive access. The Motion Pictures artists met weekly in the art studio of Norwood Crossing. She felt "honored to witness their bravery and their drive to share their visions through drawing, even though the project challenged them physically and emotionally."

Award winner Laura Evonne Steinman created a project in which participants put together artist books using a variety of materials (fabric, wood, photos, colored paper, and printed materials), books about their lives, their stories, their passions. "It's about us coming together and the books being the springboard for dialogue between all of us. We share stories while we're making these books. These people know so much and have done so much."

The potential for such projects was summed up by Randy Vick, professor in the Art Education and Art Therapy Department at the School of the Art Institute: "Art can be important to people of any age, but for seniors a lot of the value can come around things like life review, the potential for socializing and the joy of being productive… Art is wonderful way to re-engage because you see a product, and that can be very gratifying."

Our hope is that these projects will serve as models for other such efforts.

The Legacy Continues: A Play and a Film

To help tell this story even more widely, the Hilgos Foundation has developed a short play for young students, based on the concept that children will respond to a story if they actually participate in telling it. The play can be used to open a longer discussion in classrooms, in day care centers, in assisted living facilities, and with community groups who are interested in these issues.[6]

The Hilgos Foundation has also sponsored a documentary film called *I Remember Better When I Paint*, which examines the importance of art for persons afflicted with Alzheimer's and other memory disorders.[7] Narrated by actress Olivia de Havilland, it looks at this topic from the viewpoint of neurologists, researchers, physicians, art museum directors, care providers, and artists.[8]

The film shows the remarkable progress that has been made in understanding how the arts help people with Alzheimer's. When the art students first coaxed Hilgos to pick up her paintbrush and use her art to express herself and communicate with her loved ones, their work was groundbreaking. Today caregivers around the world are learning that the creative arts can tap memory and reawaken a sense of personality, identity, and dignity.

---

6   The play is described in greater detail in Chapter 13.

7   Important quotations from the film are in Chapter 12. The film is described in greater detail in Chapter 13.

8   Thank you to Mary Louise Stott, who introduced me to Eric Ellena of French Connection Films. Eric generously co-directed the film with me and Mary Louise became the associate producer.

6 The Hidden Hour

Jenny Graf Sheppard

...she painted a continuous pattern of colorful strokes. Scrutinizing her work on the page for a long while she said, with a pleased expression, "The Hidden Hour." Puzzled, I asked her to repeat herself. She looked at me and repeated, "The Hidden Hour," while placing a hand on the painting, smudging some of the paint.

That was the most I had heard Hilda say since working with her. I felt incredibly elated. Not only did she seem pleased with her own work, but she had bridged a silent gap that had existed between us."

It was late August 1995, a month before my first semester of the Masters in Fine Arts program at the School of the Art Institute of Chicago, and I had arrived early from New York to find a part-time job. I was attending graduate school to continue working with the subject of aging, memory, and identity in video and sound installations. I did not expect to find employment in the very situation I sought for my artwork. But there it was, the notice on the Art Institute job board: "I am looking for someone to paint with my mother, a 91-year-old artist, who resides in a nursing home." Excited, I phoned the number on the ad from the payphone at school. After meeting Berna, Hilda's daughter, and her father, who himself had recently moved into a retirement facility, things were settled. I was to visit Hilda three times a week for several hours at a time to paint and visit with her.

When I arrived at the convalescent home and was introduced to the staff, I explained what it was Hilda and I would be doing several hours a week. Then I went upstairs to meet Hilda. I couldn't really make any judgments about her memory or her person because Hilda would not speak. She seemed removed, and, although she had a hint of a smile, I could sense that it was for my sake, not hers. So those first weeks led me to believe that Hilda was a passive, soft-spoken person with little on her mind, due to Alzheimer's, and not much interest in interacting with me or anyone else.

When I took the watercolors out and set up the table for painting, Hilda showed no response, even when I offered her the brush. For an hour, I sat painting a bit, trying to hand off the brush to her with no success and awkwardly holding up a one-way conversation. Although I could see by the paintings in her room from decades past that she had once had a passionate relationship with the medium and with life, I decided that Hilda was no longer productive, that she was, like many other people her age, just sort of waiting in limbo. Even so, I continued to try to engage her. For the next month and a half, I saw no progress. I met with her two or three times a week but could not get her to interact, to look at me, or to paint. But then, in early October, she gradually began to respond.

The First Painting

The first painting Hilda completed while she was with me was "The Hidden Hour." For the previous two weeks I had been painting a stroke, handing her the brush to let her add something, painting a stroke again, trying to gradually step more and more out of the picture. While we worked, Hilda appeared generally uninterested and annoyed at my persistence. I wondered if what I was forcing upon her was cruel. Her attention was not directed toward the act of painting, and she seemed to be masking a hidden anger with her silence. "You do it!" Hilda seemed to be saying emphatically.

I wondered if perhaps she wasn't assuming the role of a teacher and that I was to play along as the student. Following her direction, I decided to let myself become the student, if that was what was enabling her to participate in the construction of something. I think, perhaps, it was in this role-playing, with Hilda as the teacher and me as the student, that she began to act.

Sure, this might have been trickery, but by following her lead, I gained some things as well. For one, I'd been facing a creative block with my own work, which prevented me from approaching any sort of "blank canvas." Watching her method of working was for me invaluable. In retrospect, I see that it was the decision to become her student that was a first step in subverting the limitations posed by the patient-caregiver dynamic. What was also opened up was the way for a different kind of relationship.

The day she began to paint what was to become "The Hidden Hour," Hilda worked alone without handing the brush back to me.

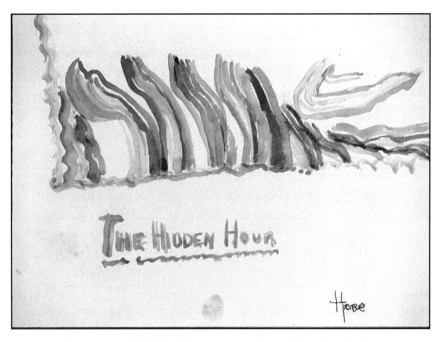

In the fall of 1995, after two months of showing little response to Jenny's efforts to paint with her, Hilgos took up the brush and created *The Hidden Hour.*

She painted a continuous pattern of colorful strokes. Scrutinizing her work on the page for a long while she said, with a pleased expression, "The Hidden Hour." Puzzled, I asked her to repeat herself. She looked at me and repeated, "The Hidden Hour," while placing a hand on the painting, smudging some of the paint.

That was the most I had heard Hilda say since I began working with her. I felt incredibly elated. Not only did she seem pleased with her own work, but she had bridged a silent gap that had existed between us. Until then I had, as one might with a young child, left open the possibility that some of her gestures and movements held a secret meaning. Even though I thought there might be more to Hilda than I knew, I could not be sure. After all, the director of the convalescent home had told me one day, "With these people the light is either on or off, and with Hilda it is definitely off." The head nurse, several weeks later, had even suggested that I not come anymore. Some of the staff had said, "She's far gone. She doesn't know what she is doing," and "You can't get her to paint. I don't know why Berna wants her to do this."

"It is true," I thought. Except for that one moment of seeming recognition, Hilda did seem far away. Berna called her every day, asking about her painting, the weather in Chicago, and her visitors. While the nurse held the receiver to her ear, Hilda sat silent, staring into space.

Despite the success of Hilda's painting "The Hidden Hour," I continued to struggle to communicate with her. It was as if, in trying to communicate, I would have to believe that there was some tangible consciousness that I was addressing and responding to. I wanted to believe that there was a level of meaning in the actions, paintings, and fragmented speech of this 91-year-old woman. "The Hidden Hour" opened up an inkling of this possibility, but it hardly carried me through the following weeks of Hilda's ongoing lack of interaction. To add to my wariness of working with her, Hilda's moods fluctuated, and I was unfamiliar with this common Alzheimer's trait.

A Breakthrough

Then one day, a few weeks later, something astonishing happened.
I prepared to leave the nursing home after another failed attempt at
involving Hilda in painting. After washing the brushes, I stopped
to say goodbye to Hilda, who was sitting in her wheelchair in the
hallway. As I turned to leave, I saw her lift up a finger, gesturing
me to come toward her. I approached her, and she offered me her
hand. I grabbed it, and she said, "I have never had anything like this
with someone, ya know?" Stunned, I nodded silently. After quite a
while, she added, "I just want to keep it this way."

Shock prevented me from knowing how to respond. With
excitement that was uncontainable, I rode my bike all the way home
grinning, completely exhilarated. My faith in the human capacity
was validated, and the part of me that was beginning to doubt what
we were doing was put to rest. I wrote her words down as soon as I
got home and sent them to her son, Leonard.

One thing I should explain is that I remember finding the
added "ya know" on the sentence comedic. It made me chuckle
silently when she said it. My friends have always poked fun at me
for my excessive use of "ya know" at the ends of sentences. And I
had been ultra-conscious of using it with Hilda, who would never
respond or nod in return. Often it would hang in the air like a
resonating bell, painfully reminding me of the chasm between
us. When Hilda used this phrase in her own sentence, it almost
convinced me that she was parroting me, not merely reflecting me
in an imitative way, but perhaps attempting to communicate using
a shared language. Hilda's comment affirmed her cognitive presence
and presented a possibility for a shared language. If we could build
our own language of meaning within our small setting, however
irrelevant that language was to the greater world, we might survive.

Hilda's Continuing Transformation

By the time a year had gone by, three other young artists from the
Art Institute were working with Hilda to provide her with daily
artistic and social activity. We had been through a lot as a group.
It was often a struggle to defend our presence there. We had all

witnessed Hilda emerge from her shell and settle into a place where she could freely articulate thoughts, albeit often in cryptic ways.

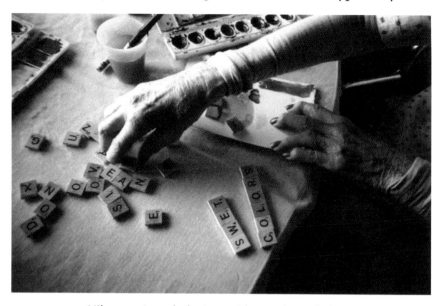

Hilgos enjoyed playing with words and ideas,
as she does here with "swet colors."

Yet, the more I learned about Hilda, the easier it was to locate her words and images in the context of who she was and who she was becoming.

For example, she went through a phase in which she would write her name in cursive over and over on a piece of paper. This activity emerged out of her deteriorating ability to sign her name at the bottom of her paintings, a skill that she had retained until recently, despite her declining memory. Noting this, we began to urge her to practice signing her artist name, Hilgos, the name she had chosen for herself and which was bound up with her artist persona. She seemed to respond to this exercise with enthusiasm, and it carried her work in a new direction. The signatures would continue religiously across the page, with no break in the line, gradually metamorphosing into other cursive-type lines such as waves, writing, writing-like lines, and loops. To me, these lines came to resemble a complex mapping of who Hilda was beyond the simple signature, a mapping composed of her love for the horizon

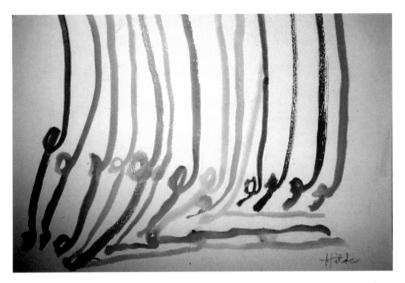

Hilgos enthusiastically extended her signature into cursive-like
lines that included waves and loops (1997).

line and for the sea, but also composed of vestiges of a signature
and a continuous line across the page that could testify to her
unfailing attention.

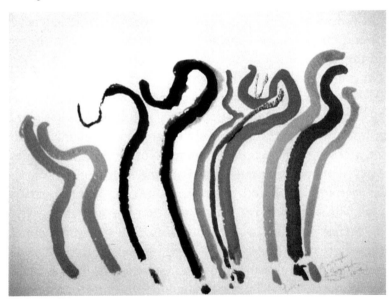

Hilgos also used cursive-like lines in a
1997 painting she named *Hilograph*.

When she used similar lines to create a painting and named it "Hilograph," it struck me as significant. On the bottom right corner, in ink, she also signed it "Hilograph." Hilda, many years ago, aware of assumptions about associations between gender and artistic authorship, dealt with this problem by using a gender-ambiguous name. The name change, in which she combined her first and last name, may have been Hilda's first attempt at authoring her public artist persona. I saw the Hilograph painting as a tongue-in-cheek extension of this: a "graph" being an image onto which measured values are projected and a "graph" as something drawn or written.

I wondered if Hilda was responding to those of us around her who were using painting as a basis for judging her capacity. There

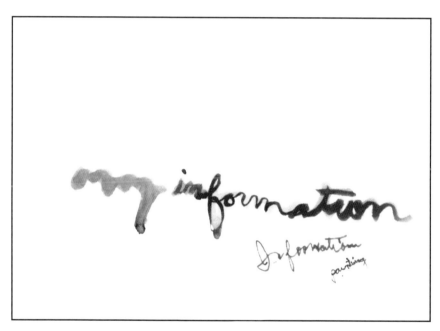

Hilgos showed she was aware that her paintings were a tool to convey information about herself (1997).

were other gestures of this sort where she seemed to be reflecting on painting as a tool to convey information about herself. For example, one work consisted solely of the painted words "My Information" and for a signature, "Information Painting." In another work, she painted the words "Done by Hilda." When asked to name the show that would feature her latest paintings and those of the art students working with her as well as my own video work about our interactions, Hilda came up with "Accessible: A Show." She was aware that by this time it was the painting that made her current relationship with the world accessible.

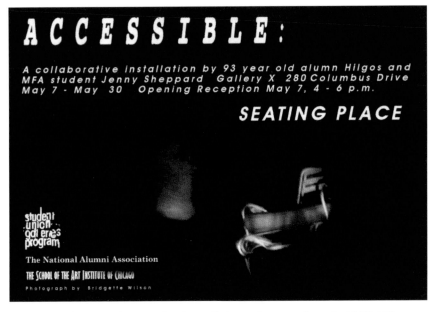

When Hilgos and Jenny had a collaborative art show in1997, Hilgos named it *Accessible,* declaring "I've never been this accessible."

Many of our innovations in working with Hilda came from listening to Hilda herself. Helen, one of Hilda's nurses who took a special interest in maintaining Hilda's creative mobility, started playing catch with her. Helen noticed that this activity had a positive effect on Hilda's mood and alertness. When we weren't there to assist with painting, Helen would take out the paints to generate Hilda's interest. Despite her lack of training, Helen would make paintings herself while Hilda looked on. These paintings would often end up on the walls alongside Hilda's own work. It was a group effort that required understanding by all.

At times, I saw the paintings Hilda made as records of actions and experiences. And I began to think of Hilda as more of a dancer than a painter. Tim[1] must have too because he made an oil painting of her in a wheelchair, wearing toe shoes. Hilda's paintings functioned like action paintings—a record of what occurred in real time. Often I felt that Hilda was more aware of concepts like these than was I—although I was an M.F.A. student in the Time Arts![2] Hilda consistently pushed my imagination about what kind of work was being accomplished and the different creative approaches I might take within my own work.

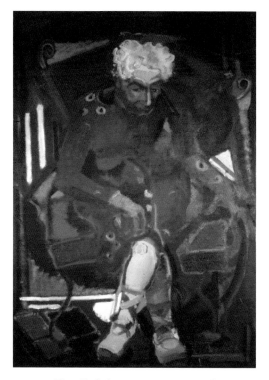

Tim Daly's 1996 painting of Hilgos in toe shoes

Sometimes her approaches would dovetail with what has been deemed to be typically Alzheimer's-like behavior. For example, Hilda would play with the objects of our paint setup, such as the various cups of water for the different brushes. She would pour the water from one cup into another, over and over. I would bring extra containers because she seemed to enjoy fitting them into each other. At times she would repeatedly get up and sit down in her chair, sometimes insisting on switching seats with me.

Another activity she enjoyed in the midst of creating work was tracing around the table at which we sat. Pinching the edge of the

---

1   Tim Daly was another art student who worked with Hilda.

2   The Time Arts program involves art that has a durational dimension. Time-based media are usually video, slide, film, audio, or computer programs. The art is experienced by watching it unfold over time as it is played back.

table with the fingers of both hands, she would walk purposefully all the way around until she arrived at the spot where she began. She once remarked, after performing this action, "That's a very fine experience."

We saw actions like these as a means for her to access creativity, but also as her way of defining spaces and examining them. Her examinations of space came through in the paintings, which at times showed signs of such investigations of edges, vessels, and volume. I think we all sensed that these were investigations of her new cognitive place in being. Another time she said, referring to

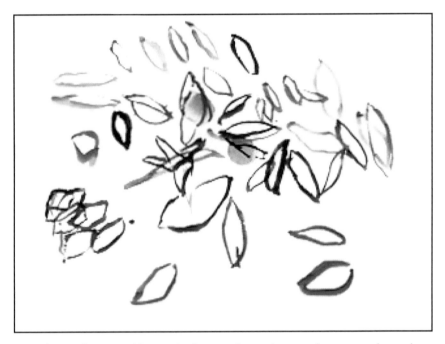

Hilgos often used her paintings to investigate edges, vessels, and volume, as shown in this 1996 painting of boat tops.

a painting she was working on made up of circular bands of color, "That's a whole defined. That's defining it."

"Would you like a cookie?" one of us had once asked.

"Yes, I'll define it," she said, taking the cookie, and she proceeded to bite speedily around its circumference.

With our daily visits, Hilda was becoming a social woman. One thing I began to notice was a change in her use of language. Typically, every few days, Hilda would speak a short sentence. Other than that, she remained quiet. Over time, we all noticed Hilda becoming freer with speech, even though her words were often hard to decipher. We would incorporate her words into our conversations so as to unravel her intricate plays on meaning. Such was the way we constructed meaning together.

The Meaning of Hilda's Transformation

Our experience as a group, documented in the paintings themselves, is an example of the progress and growth a person can experience in spite of aging, memory loss, deteriorating health, and life in a nursing home. It is assumed that a person with memory loss cannot mean what she says; thus artistic intent is called into question. Hilda's late work, however, reflects a continuation of her early themes and also presents new themes specific to her changed cognitive state. As with any great artwork, interpreting the themes in Hilda's work requires something of us too.

Once the connections can be seen between who she became and her work, it may become possible to see the high-functioning intellect that was at work behind the paintings she made in her last couple of years. The enjoyment and productivity that Hilda experienced from age 91 to 93 might be easily attributed to the people who surrounded her during this time. For me, though, the factor in all of this that really made it work was Hilda herself. Knowing that Anne Morrow Lindbergh's *A Gift from the Sea* was a book she had once treasured, I brought in a copy for her to browse through. Once again I was surprised, this time by the aptness of the passage she chose to read. It really spoke to Hilda's adaptation to her new place in the world:

*All living relationships are in process of change, of expansion,
and must perpetually be building themselves new forms.
But there is no single fixed form to express such a changing
relationship. There are perhaps different forms for each*

> *successive stage; different shells I might put in a row on my desk to suggest the different stages of marriage—or indeed of any relationship.*[3]

Hilda, in her changing cognitive states, was forming a new relationship with the world.

Jenny Graf Sheppard received her MFA in Time Arts in 1998 from the School of the Art Institute of Chicago. She is an artist and professor living in Baltimore, Maryland.

---

3   Lindbergh, Anne Morrow. *A Gift from the Sea*. New York: Pantheon Books, 2005

7 The Invincible Circle

Timothy Daly

> *The experience with Hilda deepened my
> trust in the arts as an important form of
> communication. It is very hard to predict
> a situation using the "what if . . ." concept,
> but if Hilda did not have the availability of
> art as an opportunity to communicate, she
> may not have been able to express verbally
> all of the amazing statements she so clearly
> painted.*

My first encounter with Hilda Gorenstein was a shocking one.
Here was a frail and innocent-looking, sweet, elderly woman:
a stranger to me. Her arm was wrapped in a cast as she tried
to muster herself free from two nurse's aides, seemingly out of
frustration. I approached her and almost immediately her facial
expression changed into a sweetness beyond a blossoming flower.
"Well...and how are you?" she seemed to say. I was baffled by
the metamorphosis as I helped her up from her wheelchair. My
experience working with Hilda was truly amazing. Here was a
woman who could have easily let her illness take its course, but
instead chose to build an incredible city of fresh new feelings and
vivid visual ideas.

I think the most vital aspect of working with Hilda was being
able to communicate with her. I don't mean, "Hello, how are you
today?" I mean using different means or approaches to allow her
to release what she needed to at that particular moment. Because
of her gradual memory loss brought on by Alzheimer's, Hilda had
a struggle to focus on one thing. Within this apparent confusion, I
think we as the art students provided her with a constant focus on

painting. In a sense, visual communication gave her a steady focus. I let her say whatever she needed to say at any given moment, both verbally and visually. Sometimes it was clear as the summer sky and at other times it was abstract and floating. I had to become an unbiased receptor.

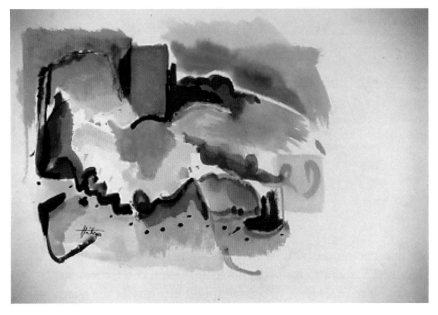

Painting was Hilgos's means of visual communication, and it gave her a steady focus (1998).

Working with Hilda was not free of obstacles. One of the main hurdles was that the nursing home was not inviting at times. Circumstances arose that prevented me from seeing her on my own terms. I was used to signing in at the front desk and riding the elevator to Hilda's floor. It would always be a treat for me to see Hilda's face light up when I entered the room, as I always surprised her. Unfortunately, I became "restricted" to the sun room, which was located on the top floor. I was told that I had been distracting other residents. It became somewhat of a hassle to visit Hilda, all the way up until she passed away. But, it did not deter me. I came every day for two hours. Those two hours I came to treasure, as I was constantly amazed and introduced to wonderful experiences.

Working with someone who had been down a long road, full of lively experiences, was an immeasurable gift to me. I remember the first time I visited Hillie's house in Highland Park and was amazed at the tranquility that it possessed. I became familiar with the numerous sculpted bodhisattvas and lamps. Seeing these pieces made me understand her graceful and poetic movements and personality. Also, seeing her earlier works allowed me to clearly connect her continual interest in the horizon and ocean life.

I was not the only one who visited Hilda. Jenny Sheppard was the first to begin to work with Hilda. Jenny really helped me a lot with her own insights. Jane Benson and Robin Barcus-Slonina also worked with Hilda, and they brought in yet another set of terrific observations. We all formed an invincible circle of support in which Hilda could dance. Berna, Hilda's daughter, was tremendous throughout the whole time I worked with Hilda. She would always send postcards and letters. Every day, Berna would call and ask how

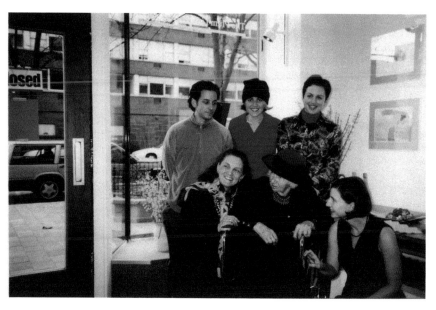

The invincible circle of support for Hilgos included Berna Huebner and Robin Barcus-Slonina (front row with Hilda), and Tim Daly, Jenny Sheppard, and Jane Benson (back row). They are attending a gallery showing of Hilda's artwork.

"Mom" was doing. Berna, Jenny, Robin, Jane, and Hilda—they all became an extended family to me.

My main goal was to give Hilda a structure in which she could express her ideas: a blank piece of paper and a paintbrush. I think there was a great deal of communication that occurred in Hilda's late body of work that might not have been expressed without the vehicle of visual art. I have always seen art as a means to communicate with others. Being an artist means that you are continually setting up a dialogue with yourself and your audience. Through visual language it is often possible to speak more forcefully than you can with words. I believe that all great works of art possess this incredible non-verbal power. When I see a Van Gogh from across the room in a museum, I am inexorably drawn to its inexplicable intensity. To try to describe some feelings with words seems useless to me, and that is why I make paintings: so people can see and experience them.

I also enjoyed accompanying Hilda to museums. Usually one of the other art students came with us, or sometimes Berna and

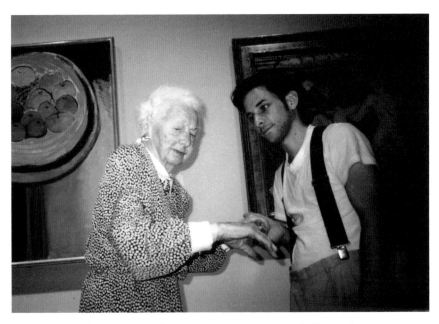

Hilgos enjoyed going to museums and discussing the paintings with Tim and the other art students.

her sons, David and Charley. Hilda especially loved to focus on Turner's marine paintings at the Art Institute of Chicago. She could sit for a long time just looking at his paintings with waves and at other Turner paintings. One could see how calm she became just looking. She also enjoyed discussing paintings with us. We also accompanied Hilda to other museums—one of her own paintings was exhibited at the Spertus Museum on Michigan Avenue. Looking at and talking about paintings helped her communicate and connect with us. All of us enjoyed these outings.

The experience of working with Hilda taught me numerous things. It introduced me to the concept of patience. Being a visual artist, one has to possess patience in order to create. Waiting or just letting ideas come in and out without passing judgment is a challenge, but it is a vital part of the artistic process. Through working with Hilda, I developed a unique kind of patience. Her nurses also taught me about patience. They were tremendously good at understanding her particular situation and assessing her needs at all times. Their patience and consistency were essential to Hilda's life.

The experience with Hilda also deepened my trust in the arts as an important form of communication. Although it is very hard to predict a situation using the "what if ..." concept, if Hilda did not have the availability of art as a means to communicate, she may not have been able to express in any other way all of the amazing thoughts and emotions she so clearly painted.

As I write this, I have just begun my career as a teacher. I am currently substitute-teaching in the New York City Public Schools. I believe that it is the teacher's responsibility—in fact, duty—to bring the information to the kids in an exciting, consistent, and fresh way. One has to assess the situation and follow the individual flow of the classroom. To think that there is a universal syllabus that will work for everyone is foolish. The same idea applied to working with Hilda. Some days we painted, some days we talked, and some days we just sat together.

The invincible circle that connected all of us who worked with Hilda has yet to be broken. Together we created a scholarship fund for those who wish to pursue jobs with a similar art-related structure. From 1995 to 1998, we organized a series of exhibitions of Hilda's work, and I've been busy making molds of Hilda's sculptures and casting them to be sold to benefit the scholarship fund.

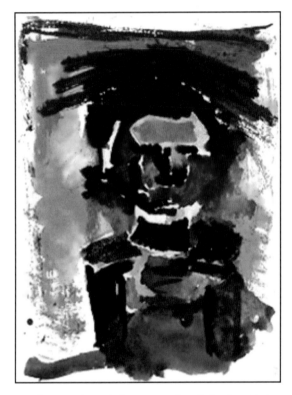

Hilgos painted this portrait of Tim in1996.

Throughout the two years I worked with Hilda, I learned a tremendous amount. Each day was always new and interesting. I became quite close to her, as did Jenny, Jane, and Robin, and it was difficult to see her pass. Still I think of her often and apply the skills I've gained. I feel very fortunate to have worked with her. I always feel warm inside when I think about Hilda and the precious time I spent with her and our poignant talks on art.

I will close with a remark that Hilda once made. I had brought in my George Braque book for Hilda to look at. She gazed at the painting titled "The Boat" (1960) and remarked, "This one has a story and a remembrance. These things are good and it makes it worthwhile."

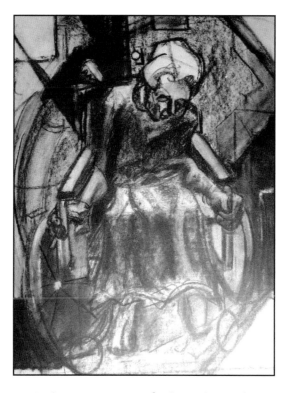

Tim's 1996 portrait of Hilgos shows the
beauty and grace he saw in her.

Timothy J.Daly received his BFA from the School of the Art Institute (SAIC) in 1998. He was awarded an SAIC scholarship to study painting and drawing at Lorenzo De'Medici in Florence, Italy (Fall of 1996). He is a working artist currently living in Brooklyn, NY. He has helped many international artists fabricate small- and large-scale public works.

8 Hitting a Different Spot

Jane Benson

> *By painting, Hilda continued to connect
> with those around her.*

During the time I was working with Hilda, she found inspiration
for the paintings she produced in postcards and photographs.
The many and varied images were sent to her primarily by her
daughter Berna and were vital to Hilda's production. Full of vibrant
colors and inspirational forms, the postcards were also warm with
an intense emotional energy that awakened Hilda's appetite for
painting and communicating.

At first, Hilda would sit down at the beginning of our
afternoons together and instinctively start painting directly onto
the face of the postcard or photograph chosen for the day. Rather
than using them as the source for inspiration, interpretation was
side-stepped. The image became the source, the subject matter, and
the artwork. Both cause and effect were enmeshed. Painting on
the photograph and over the image created an intensely beautiful
and complex image. The colors always complemented those in the
image, while partially obscuring and changing the reality originally
captured in the photograph.

No interpretation was necessary on Hilda's behalf to create the
painted postcards. What became apparent, after many a day had
commenced with producing these idiosyncratic works, was how
they opened a door to the complicated, multi-layered relationship
existing between the real and the representational, not only in
Hilda's work, but in her life.

Hilda's reality appeared to those around her like a representation of reality, a reinvented reality. Similar to the representation that existed in the painted postcards, hers was a filtered reality, obscured and complicated by a mind that possessed the power to morph memory and a conventional sense of things.

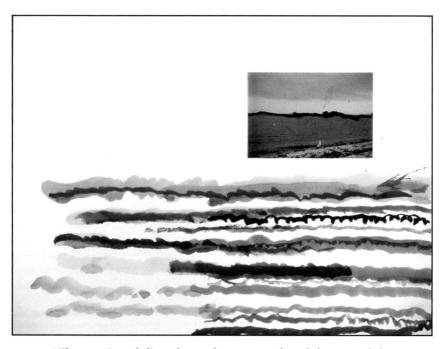

Hilgos painted directly on the postcard and then used the colors and lines to inspire her own expression (1996).

I housed a deep affection and admiration for these altered postcards, but worked with Hilda to change direction and start painting on the awaiting piece of watercolor paper that stared blankly at both of us. We worked together against the instinct—the Alzheimer's instinct—that produced the painted postcards, and instead, guided her thoughts and gentle hand towards the thirsty paper. Making this change frequently marked a transition in Hilda's mood. She would spend longer on these paintings and grow calmer during their production. When Hilda placed the paintbrushes on the table, a gesture that marked the completion of a painting, there would be a sense of clarity and peacefulness to her demeanor.

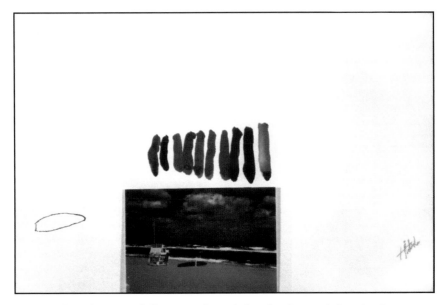

Hilgos has carefully reproduced the shades and tints in the postcard and has also reproduced the shape of the boat (1996).

Hilda's relationship with her surroundings became increasingly physical as her ability to communicate through words declined. Touch and sight were central to communication. They were the tools employed to paint. By painting, Hilda continued to connect with those around her. The complexity of her interpretation of reality and her ability to express how she experienced that reality through color and form enabled her to continue to be active within her changing world. The opportunity to reach others through her work, to share thoughts and emotions evoked by the paintings, worked like a charm to raise Hilda's spirits. This exchange restored the sparkle in her eye and in all the loving eyes around her.

I was always told how powerful and thoroughly full of life Hilda had been, creating rich and vibrant relationships with all who shared her life. Her work of this period revealed that her relationship with her surroundings had reached new, intricate, and complex levels of understanding. Hilda's frames of reference may have been depleted, reality obscured by a mind losing memory; however, the watercolor paintings, and in particular the painted postcards, shed light on the ever-changing and unique relationship she had with the world.

Jane Benson was born in England and moved to the US on a Fulbright Scholarship in 1995. She received her BA from Edinburgh College of Art (1994) and her MFA from the School of The Art Institute of Chicago (1997). A multidisciplinary artist, Jane Benson now lives and works in New York. She is currently represented by Thierry Goldberg Projects, New York and continues to show her work nationally and internationally.

9 Hilda: A Jewel Distilled

Robin Barcus-Slonina

> *By far the biggest lesson I learned in my time with Hilda is that the creative process is as essential to an artist as breathing, especially after it has been cultivated over the course of an entire lifetime. This was certainly true of Hilda and remained true, regardless of her deteriorating health.*

I had the good fortune of knowing and working with Hilda Gorenstein for two years, a mere fraction of the 93 she spent as a creative presence in this world. Hilda was a prolific artist her whole life, enjoying a successful career as a nautical painter commissioned to paint sea vessels. Her paintings are privately owned around the world and are also in the collection of the Spertus Museum in Chicago. A true trailblazer, Hilda was one of the first women awarded a major Works Project Administration grant in the 1930s and painted fourteen panels depicting "The History of Our Navy" for the Chicago Century of Progress Exposition.

Toward the end of her life, however, she put down her brushes as progressive memory loss attributed to Alzheimer's disease robbed her of the ability to set up her own art materials. During a particularly lucid moment, Hilda confided to her daughter, Berna Huebner, "I remember better when I paint." Upon the suggestion of geriatric physician Dr. Lawrence Lazarus, Berna contacted Hilda's alma mater, the School of the Art Institute of Chicago, to find students to work with Hilda and hopefully to inspire her to continue painting.

By the time I responded to the School's call, artists Jenny Sheppard, Tim Daly, and Jane Benson had already been working with Hilda for several months. They had made impressive progress reaching her, re-opening the channel to her crucial mode of self-expression by holding daily art sessions with her in her nursing home. The initial groundwork was laid out to the point where all I needed to do was ask, "Do you want to paint?" and the answer was invariably a spoken yes or a nod. A cup of water, watercolors, and good paper would then be placed in front of her and a brush placed in her hand.

At this point, the transformation she underwent was phenomenal. Her face lit up, and eyes that may have been wandering aimlessly around the room came into clear, focused concentration. Expertly she would dip her brush into the water, twirling the tip against the edge of the cup to remove any excess moisture, then move over to the paint to choose her color, often

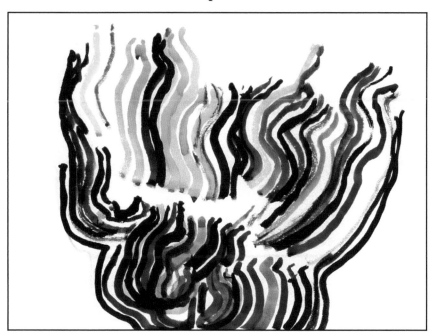

Hilgos mostly painted with the cool blues, purples, and greens that recalled her lifetime of nautical painting, as shown in *Gift of the Sea*, painted in 1997.

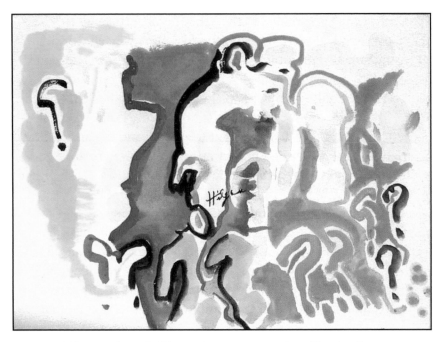

When agitated, Hilgos chose warm colors like the fiery
reds, oranges, and yellows in this 1997 painting.

using the lid of the paint set to mix her own shades. It was obvious
that Hilda had held a brush in her hand for more than seven
decades.

I noticed her color choices tended to reflect her current mood.
Mostly she used the cool blues, purples, and greens that recalled her
lifetime of nautical painting. When agitated, however, as she often
was after medical exams or baths, she chose warm colors like fiery
reds, oranges, and yellows, colors she had also used in some of her
experimental abstract paintings from the 1970s. When beginning
our sessions in an agitated mood, she might announce, "Quick,
quick!" while her materials were being set up, but the process of
painting would have a dramatic calming effect on her. She became
visibly more relaxed and peaceful, and even her breathing would
slow down.

At times, Hilda would forget the step of adding color to her
brush, and it became necessary for her assistants to do so for her.
Choosing her colors was a responsibility we all took seriously,

and fortunately by that time we had developed a sense of her preferences based on her mood and chosen subject matter. She rejected colors she did not want by pushing the brush away or dropping it unused back into the water cup. If she did begin painting with a color that didn't please her, she stopped abruptly mid-stroke and gave the brush back, usually covering the previous mark with the next color she did agree upon. On the best days, there flowed between Hilda and her assistants an unspoken understanding of her intentions, so that we felt like an extension of her, as if we were her extra arm.

Her subject matter varied greatly, but there were several major patterns into which this late work can be grouped. By far the most prevalent was a continuing exploration of her nautical themes: the sea, sky, shore, seabirds, and sailboats that she adored her whole life. The vestiges of her earlier masterful renderings of these subjects remained evident in this late work, although transformed into a new system of spontaneous personal gestures that bordered

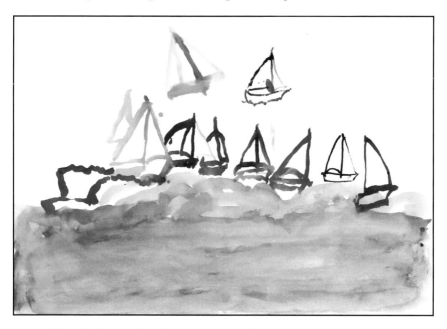

Hilgos followed the classic pattern of many great artists, which leads them further and further into abstractions of their chosen subject matter, as shown in *Sailboats*, painted in 1996.

on the abstract. While it is true that Hilda's dwindling faculties prevented her from producing the realistic depictions that she had been commissioned to make in the past, she was nonetheless following the classic pattern of many great artists. Typically, the artistic career of most painters, including Matisse, Picasso, and Monet, leads them further and further into abstractions of their chosen subject matter.

Two other major groups of Hilda's late work were line and circle paintings, arguably the two most basic shapes in the language of visual depiction. Repetitive, waving lines seemed another reference to water, and the circles had a particularly soothing effect on Hilda, like the mandalas[1] representing "wholeness" or "self" in Jungian psychology. The repetitive action of layering lines or circles of wet color seemed particularly satisfying to Hilda, while the effort

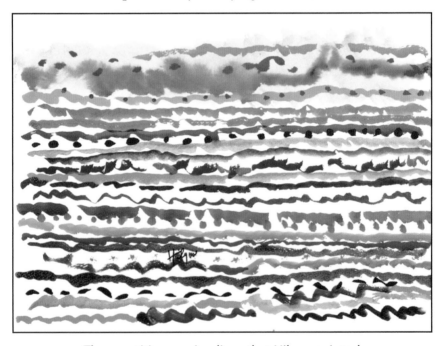

The repetitive, waving lines that Hilgos painted
seemed another reference to water (1997).

---

1   Mandalas are ritualistic geometric designs symbolic of the universe. In addition to their use in Jungian psychology, they are used in Hinduism and Buddhism as an aid to meditation.

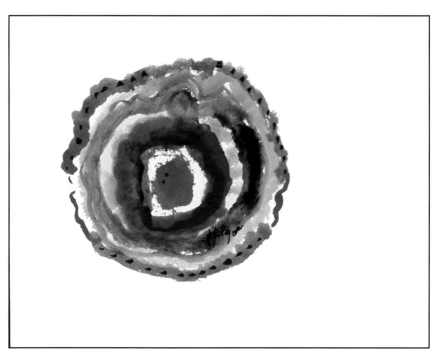

Painting circles had a particularly soothing effect on Hilgos (1997).

and concentration it demanded focused her sharp mind, which at times had difficulty expressing itself in any other way. Even in these apparently simple compositions, which brought to mind the uncomplicated eloquence of Asian art that Hilda had been fond of, the trained eyes of the artists who worked with her found the color choices and placement of compositional elements strikingly accomplished.

At times, Hilda became so relaxed while painting that she fell asleep, taking little catnaps of several minutes, then immediately resuming her painting upon awakening. During these naps, I took the opportunity to sketch Hilda, as her beauty and the deep lines etched into her face irresistibly lent themselves to blind contour drawing, a method whereby the artist keeps her eyes on the subject she is depicting without glancing down at the paper. It is a technique art students are taught to increase their observational skills without being distracted by self-conscious concern over the

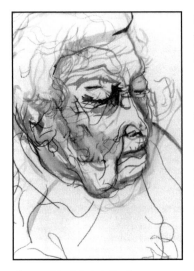

One of Robin's blind contour drawing of Hilgos (1997)

resulting image. Although my student years were behind me, it had become my favorite way to draw.

After my first year of working with Hilda, I had completed so many of these drawings that an exhibition was organized at the Plum Line Gallery in Evanston, showing Hilda's paintings alongside my portraits of her. This show was a great success, attracting publicity and attention to Hilda's situation. She attended the exhibition and smiled at everyone from her wheelchair, dressed up in one of her favorite hats.

Someone close to Hilda approached me that night and asked how long I had known her. When I replied one year, he seemed perplexed.

"I don't understand," he said. "These drawings of yours show her how she used to be, as if you knew her before."

"She is still here!" I assured him, but was met with only an expression that showed his doubt and the pain of missing what he felt was already lost.

It is true that her past was a lot to live up to. She was a phenomenal woman and a beloved wife and mother. In addition to her artistic accomplishments, she was an independent, stylish, and intelligent woman who raced sailboats on Lake Michigan and in the Atlantic Ocean. She did not let societal prejudice stand in her way, even though she felt it necessary at the time to change her professional name, signing her work with the more androgynous persona of "Hilgos." It is because of women like Hilda, who came before us, that women of my generation can so easily take our art careers for granted. She was creative in whatever she did, whether she was painting, sculpting lamps, or helping her children mold clay seashells directly onto the walls of their entrance hall at home.

By far the biggest lesson I learned in my time with Hilda is that the creative process is as essential to an artist as breathing, especially after it has been cultivated over the course of an entire lifetime. This was certainly true of Hilda, and it remained true, regardless of her deteriorating health.

Precisely because we had not known her before, the artists who worked with Hilda had no shared personal history that prevented us from seeing her in anything but her present light. We did not relate to her in terms of what was lost, but responded to her wholly based on her current state. What we found was a creative, strong, and very funny woman, whose illness had undeniably stripped her of some faculties and functions. However, the shedding of those layers of "normality" did not make her any less human in our eyes, but even more so. There was a purity of existence in her present condition that was movingly spiritual, while still punctuated by flashes of the spunk, drive, ironic humor, and sharp intellect of the woman she was, albeit now traveling through a labyrinth of mental processes to emerge. Once, when asked if she could hear

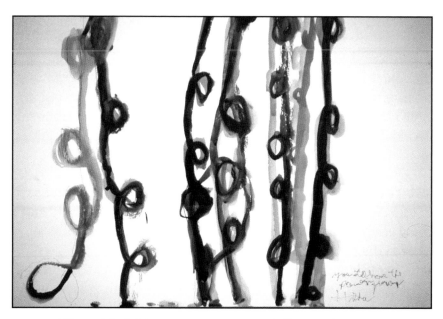

Hilgos titled this 1997 painting *You Still Have the Power,*
indicating her sense of her own power.

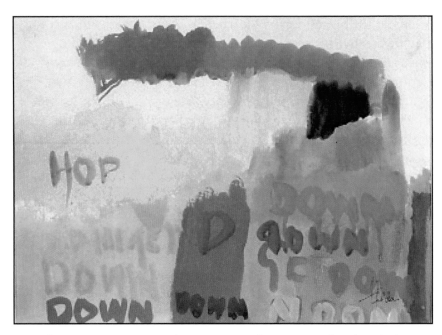

Text became an increasingly important element in Hilgos's painting as she incorporated repeated thoughts or snatches of conversation (1997).

the birds singing outside of her window, she responded, "Yes, and I can hear them talking, too." When asked what they were saying, she answered blithely, "Oh, just the usual things people say during the course of the day." Some cynics might call this nonsense, but perhaps the ability to hear birds "talking" and to experience visions, which she would occasionally describe, is nature's compensation for loss, and could even be seen, conversely, in terms of what is gained by the diseased or mentally ill.

One of the wonderful things about spending time with Hilda was the opportunity to enter into her distinct and peculiar mode of verbal communication. At times, Hilda was startlingly lucid and could easily hold what society considers a "normal" conversation. Most of the time that I knew her, however, her speech had transformed into an abstract, poetic conveyance of her thoughts, using words that could be baffling but always intriguing as we attempted to trace her threads of meaning. Often, we simply flowed with her peculiar logic and would hold absurdist dialogues with

Hilda, which were, nevertheless, steeped in humor, irony, and original ideas.

In her youth, Hilda dabbled in fashion design and illustration, and her sense of personal style never left her. Whenever I arrived wearing a hat that struck her fancy, she immediately tried it on. One winter I was carrying a vintage beaded purse I had bought second-hand, and anytime she saw it, she insisted it was hers. I thought perhaps she had once owned a similar bag, so one day I opened it to show her that this one contained my things.

"Hmm, just as I thought," she said, poking a finger through my possessions, "It's mine, all mine." And she snapped the purse shut and tucked it under her arm. Needless to say, I dumped my stuff in a plastic bag and the purse became hers!

Another faculty that did not diminish with time was Hilda's perfect eyesight, which I must admit was superior to my own. She used this to aid her habit of pulling words from the most obscure sources, reading a sign across the room, for example, and

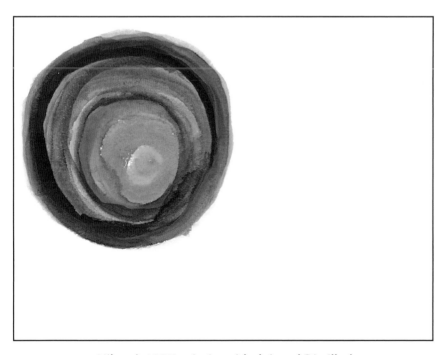

Hilgos's 1997 painting titled *Jewel Distilled*

incorporating what she had read into a sentence. To get at her meaning at times involved a visual treasure hunt for text around the room. Text became an increasingly important element of her painting as well, as she incorporated repeated thoughts or snatches of conversation around her into her painting. She might also take one word and play with derivations of it in luminous color across an entire page: "king, kin, pin, ping."

Hilda was equally creative when titling her work. One day she had just completed a beautiful circle painting with layers of shimmering color, which she seemed particularly pleased with, and I asked her what she would like to title it. She held out her fingers, bent with age and arthritis yet still skillful and strong, and placed them in the center of the circle she had just painted.

"Jewel Distilled," she announced.

"Wow," I thought, "how appropriate," and rushed to write the title and date on the back of the painting. Only later in the afternoon did I realize that there was a bottle of "distilled" water from "Jewel," a food store, directly in front of her on the table. Was the significance drawn from this mundane source just a lucky coincidence, or a conscious application of meaning gleaned from an increasingly confusing jumble of stimuli around her? Either way, I laughed out loud and pointed to the bottle.

"Jewel distilled, huh?" I asked her.

She chuckled and gave me one of her typical half-smiles, which, like the Mona Lisa's, contained a wealth of mystery and meaning, potentially maddening in its apparent inaccessibility, but never less than beautiful to witness, if one takes the time to see.

Robin Barcus-Slonina, a 1993 graduate of the School of the Art Institute of Chicago, is a multidisciplinary artist who has shown her work at galleries and museums all over the world. She had the honor of painting with Hilda Gorenstein during the last years of her life and was deeply affected and inspired by their unique interaction.

Part III: Using Art and Creative Therapies

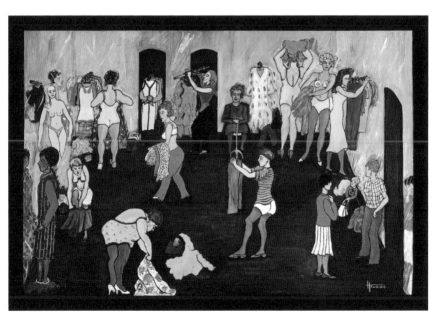

Changing Room by Hilgos, 1972

10 The Lessons of My Journey

Berna G. Huebner

Cognitive experts can help answer such questions as, "What really goes on in the brain when an artist expresses herself on canvas?"

The power of art is transformative. This is an accepted principle for young artists and a familiar reassurance for many adults. What is only now being recognized is the transformative power of art for people of all ages and, as this book has demonstrated, for those with memory loss.

In my years of work in this field, beginning with my mother and the inspiring art students from the School of the Art Institute of Chicago and continuing through my recent documentary film and this book, attitudes and awareness have changed dramatically for the better. But the transformative power of art is still inadequately understood by those afflicted with Alzheimer's and other forms of memory loss and by their families, their caregivers, and the wider medical community. There is still much to be done to educate and advocate for this approach.

Among the remaining tasks is adapting medical education to include more current information on the capabilities of art in helping the brain make new connections. As Stella Safo, a medical school student, said, "In the medical world that I dwell in as a third-year medical student at Harvard, we learn about Alzheimer's patients as those whose dementia has stolen their minds and, sadly, the quintessence of their very personalities. They remain caricatures of their original selves." This may have been an acceptable picture based on old knowledge and assumptions. But new information has been gathered. We now know more. Stella also said about my mother, "In those moments when she painted, she lived." Awareness of this possibility should be given to our new physicians and nurses.

Stella's comments echo those of Dorothy Seman, the inspirational Chicago dementia expert who wrote Chapter 11 and helped me with the resource list in Chapter 13. Dorothy stated, "I think our health education does not begin to teach the potential for the sacred/spiritual relationship that can and should exist. Much of the real comfort and healing that needs to be done is in the context of listening 'with the ears of our heart.'" In retrospect, that's what I was doing—listening with the ears of my heart—when I asked my mother if she wanted to start painting again and she gave the answer that caught my attention, inspired my action, and became the title of this book.

Another area that needs more attention is interdisciplinary work between physicians and cognition scientists.[1] Cognitive experts can help answer such questions as, "What really goes on in the brain when an artist expresses herself on canvas?" Making art is thinking. It is unproductive to approach artistic activity simply as some sort of spontaneous, unconscious "self-expression." Even the most ad hoc-looking result—a Jackson Pollock painting, for example—results from complex mental choices of, among other things, pigment, placement and, in Pollock's case, speed. We need to understand better how the brain operates during these creative acts. Because activated areas of the brain receive greater blood flow and oxygen, we should not be surprised to discover positive side-effects from an engaged, creating brain.

Moreover, we need to collect more clinical information about the real changes in patients with memory loss. As Dr. Noronha suggests in Chapter 3, before and after studies are needed of Alzheimer's patients who participate in consistent, engaged art activity.

---

1   I am indebted for this comment to Jacqueline M.F. Samuel, Ph.D., who refers readers interested in this point to Rudolph Arnheim's classic, *Art and Visual Perception: A Psychology of the Creative Eye*, revised edition, University of California Press, 1974, and Jacqueline Goodnow's book, *Children Drawing (The Developing Child)*, Harvard University Press, 1977.

But these tasks, important though they are, take a distant second place to the chilling reality that faces a person with early Alzheimer's and his/her family as the disease begins its inexorable campaign against memory. This book offers many suggestions for how families and caregivers can use art to ameliorate this reality. The lessons of my own experience suggest the following principal steps in this process:

- **Conduct a bio-psycho-social evaluation of the patient.**
  First, as Dr. Lazarus recommends in Chapter 4, a thorough bio-psycho-social evaluation of the patient should be conducted by a physician or other health professional who is open to the use of art as a constructive element in the afflicted person's life. Consideration should be given to discontinuing consultation with any medical professional who arbitrarily rejects the possibility of using the creative arts.

- **Make video and other records of the person.**
  Second, as Dr. Cohen suggests in Chapter 2, video and other records of the person should be made and preserved before the disease develops too far. These will serve both as records for the family and as a means of informing medical and nursing home staff about the patient as a functioning person, not simply as an Alzheimer's patient.

- **Connect the artistic activity with the person's past.**
  Third, connect the artistic activity with something important in the person's past. The stories in this book are about an accomplished artist, but I believe that my mother's lifelong artistic engagement was not a prerequisite for her successful experience. What is important is creative engagement, and it may take some experimentation to discover what works best. The key is that the artistic activity not be simply a time-filler. It must engage the person.

- **Get help.**

  Fourth, get help. Because consistent, persistent engagement is the key ingredient for progress and family members may not be able to stay engaged all the time, look for help outside your family. Volunteers at nursing homes and senior centers, art students as described in this book, and practicing artists in the community may be among the available resources.

- **Allow time and be persistent.**

  Fifth, be prepared for the process to take time. It is obvious from Jenny Graf Sheppard's story of working with my mother (in Chapter 6) that progress did not occur quickly or evenly. In addition, institutional skepticism may need to be overcome. Persistence is required.

- **Create a variety of activities.**

  Sixth, create a variety of activities related to the central creative process. In my mother's case, her own painting with the art students was paired with visits to museums and to familiar paintings that she had known and loved over many decades.

- **Adapt your expectations.**

  Seventh, understand the dynamics of Alzheimer's and memory loss. Adapt your expectations, painful though that may be, to the decline in lifelong capacities and satisfactions that have characterized the person. Some of the books and websites described in the resource list will help you make this difficult adjustment.

- **Know that the brain can re-wire and re-learn.**

  Eighth, learn about the growing understanding in the scientific community of the ability of the brain to re-wire and re-learn, even into advanced maturity. This astonishing attribute of the human brain is being better understood every day and explains why creative engagement in advanced years is possible, even with persons afflicted with memory loss.

It is my hope that the memoirs and essays in this book as well as the websites and books included in the resources chapter will help many patients, families, and professionals use art to restore dignity, identity, and connection for persons with memory loss. I know they can find the inspiration in their own lives like the one I heard when my mother said, "Oh yes! I remember better when I paint."

11 Now What? Including Art in Caring for Patients with Memory Loss

Dorothy Seman, R.N., M.S.

> *If a man has two pennies, he should spend one to buy a loaf of bread to sustain life and the other to buy a flower to make life worth living.*
>
> *Chinese Proverb*

One of the major challenges for the family and friends of persons with memory loss is to find ways to help diagnosed individuals to not only survive but thrive. Although the dementia causes changes and losses, many skills and interests remain intact long into the illness. The key to successful care includes understanding the unique needs, interests, and abilities of the person with dementia and adapting our approach to accommodate this.

Why Art Is Meaningful to Persons with Memory Loss

Verbal and written communication erodes over time, but meaningful communication is often still possible until the end of life. Introducing or sustaining an interest in the arts is one of the ways to maintain important feelings of connection. Engagement in art activities can serve to keep alive to one's core identity and memories, and it can re-awaken interpersonal connections with others through sharing this experience.

Persons with dementia often report intense feelings of isolation. Participating in art programs can help these persons re-engage in relationships and experience and share feelings that are an essential part of their humanity and life journeys.

Settings Where Care Is Provided

Regardless of where care is provided, art can be an important part of the overall plan of care. Although the settings may differ, there is no way to underestimate the value of art programs for the people being cared for in each of these environments. The location of care does not necessarily suggest the needs and abilities of the persons cared for. Many persons may appear detached and uninterested, but can "come alive" when others show a genuine and consistent interest in connecting with them. It is important to not be fooled by superficial appearances.

Care can be provided in a variety of settings. It can be provided in one's home or the home shared with other family members. Even as the disease progresses, many families may be able to continue care at home with the use of additional resources. This may include additional help from family, friends, and volunteers from religious groups or other community organizations. Some persons with dementia attend adult day programs that meet a variety of needs. These environments can support a diverse range of individual and group activities. Care is often provided in residential settings, such as assisted living facilities or nursing homes.

Impact of Dementia on the Activity

There are some considerations that should be taken into account when planning art activities for individuals or groups with dementia:

- **There may be a decreased ability to initiate or quickly engage in activities**. Providing a framework or structure is important. It may take a while to develop the art activity focus. Within that framework, many persons with dementia may be able to make choices about how they would like to be involved. Others may need more direction and encouragement, or they may prefer to be on the periphery of an activity, observing or involved episodically.

- **Sensory environment can be overwhelming**. Many persons with dementia have increasing difficulty managing noise and crowds. It makes it harder for them to focus and concentrate on the task at hand, often causing distress. It is essential to continually evaluate what needs to be done to maintain the comfort of all persons in the art activity.

- **Communication will be affected**. Over time, the symptoms of memory loss will affect communication in many complex ways. There may be word-finding problems and difficulty keeping up the usual pace of communication. The best approach is to be tuned in to all forms of communication, verbal as well as non-verbal. From those cues we should be accepting and adjust our response in a way that meets the person's needs and abilities.

- **Be sure that expectations are realistic**. People's needs change over time, and we must be sensitive to these fluctuations or loss of interest or ability. We must focus on the persons we are caring for and not on our needs or our sadness over a loss of sharing some activities.

- **Be sensitive to the cultural differences in art heritage and history**. American society is rapidly becoming more diverse. When developing programs for groups of persons with memory loss, we must be knowledgeable about their art history and the iconic images that are part of their heritage.

Level of Interest in the Arts

The love of art may be a central part of the personal identity of some people. This may include the creation of works of art or a deep knowledge or appreciation of art developed over a lifetime. For others, engagement with the arts may come later in life, perhaps through participation in programs after the person was diagnosed. The focus must be on understanding the needs and preferences of the person at the present moment.

Impact of Other Medical Conditions

We all age in different ways. Be sure to evaluate the person's physical health for conditions that may limit participation in art programs. The purpose here is to find ways to avoid discomfort and enable the person to be successful in art activities. Conditions such as arthritis or Parkinson's disease may cause pain or coordination difficulties. Changes in vision caused by advanced cataracts, glaucoma, macular degeneration, or color blindness may affect the ability to create or view art. Heart conditions or breathing problems may make concentration more limited.

How You Can Help the Broader Community

Despite the progress made in dementia research, many physicians and other health care professionals have a limited understanding of the impact of dementia. Some have an undue sense of futility and a lack of appreciation for the many ways to sustain people with dementia through programs that emphasize social activities. In our society today there is a prevailing focus on the medical model of care, with an emphasis on treatment of the disease and management of the symptoms. This approach limits many avenues of care. By broadening our focus to include helping individuals with memory loss to live their lives fully, we can open our minds to the many possibilities that exist to improve the quality of life.

Heighten Awareness Through Advocacy

Consider ways to share success. Sharing your enthusiasm and stories of positive experiences can often create momentum for change. Consider the following strategies and add your ideas to the growing number of ways to advance the inclusion of art in programs for persons with dementia. Don't underestimate the importance of your experience in expanding the perspectives of health care staff and other family members.

- **Share your experience** during discussions with members of the health care team who care for your family member.

- **Offer to write an article** for newsletters published by various groups with whom you interact; for example, your local Alzheimer's Association or your doctor's practice.

- **Ask the local Alzheimer's Association** to include information on using the arts in caring for people with dementia in conferences for family caregivers and health care staff.

- **Offer to do a presentation** about your successful experience in using art as part of a panel discussion at a local conference.

- **Encourage family members** who are in school to do a class project on the use of art in caring for persons with memory loss.

- **Make financial contributions or donate supplies**. Even in the best of times, there is a lack of funding to develop and sustain programs that support art as part of the therapeutic health care programs. Most programs welcome donations of money or supplies to be used to develop, enrich, or expand in-house art programs. Funds are helpful to support trips to art museums in the community, including transportation costs, parking costs, and admission fees. These trips are often very labor-intensive when trying to insure the safety and enjoyment of everyone participating in the trip.

Develop Community Programs Through Partnerships

There are enormous opportunities to stimulate program development on a small or large scale. Many of the seeds that are planted create an energy and a synergy that can have far-reaching effects and can ignite in others a passion to plan innovative programs using the arts. Each of us has a network of family, friends, neighbors, and co-workers who may be eager to support exciting new initiatives. Consider ways to identify like-minded individuals and achieve the following activities—together, if possible

- **Offer to volunteer your time and talent** to assist organizations that want to initiate or expand their use of art programs. An extra set of hands can provide individual assistance to persons with memory loss. A sustained commitment is vital because there is a learning curve involved in developing quality programs.

- **Seek ways to make substantial contributions** that can have a sustained impact on art programs:

  ⇒ The need for **transportation**, a mini-van or small bus, is often a prohibitive cost for group programs—adult day care as well as residential programs.

  ⇒ Many **colleges or universities** with health care programs do not have a degree program in therapeutic arts. Others may have an insufficient number of faculty or a lack of scholarships for students interested in a career in therapeutic recreation.

  ⇒ Some **health care facilities** cannot afford consultants to create meaningful arts programs. Others do not have funding to pay for freelance staff who could lead art groups.

  ⇒ Health care programs often do not have the **audio-visual equipment or art books** that could be used to address the wide range of interests and abilities with multi-ethnic groups of people.

Sustained initiative is needed to help develop *partnerships* between art institutes and the programs that care for people with memory loss.

Dorothy Seman is Coordinator of Home and Community-Based Programs at the Jesse Brown Veterans Administration Medical Center in Chicago. She has over 35 years of experience in working with people diagnosed with dementia and is the author of "Defining Dignity: A Means to Creative Intervention," which was published in Alzheimer's Care Today, April/June 2005 and July/September 2007 issues.

12 Additional Comments from Doctors and Caregivers

Deborah Lange

> *In spite of Alzheimer's, the essence of*
> *each person continues on, still ready to*
> *communicate, often through new paths, to*
> *touch and be touched, to love and be loved.*
> *Olivia de Havilland, Narrator*

The following comments are from the documentary film *I Remember Better When I Paint.*[1]

The Science of Alzheimer's Disease

Alzheimer's doesn't affect the entire brain all at once. It seems to selectively start in the parts of the brain that are important for laying down new memory. That's why people with Alzheimer's disease may sometimes remember things from the far past but have a great deal of difficulty learning new things.
Dr. Robert Green, Associate Director for Research, Genetic Medicine, Brigham and Women's Hospital and Harvard Medical School

There are parts of the brain that are involved much later that are involved in creativity. There's a part of the brain called the parietal lobe[2] that's involved in Alzheimer's but rather late and that part of

---

1   Co-directed by Eric Ellena and Berna Huebner and released by French Connection Films in September 2009. The film is described in greater detail in Chapter 13.

2   The parietal lobe...deals with the perception and integration of stimuli from the senses. (National Institute on Aging. *Alzheimer's Disease: Unraveling the Mystery*. 2008. p. 11)

the brain is stimulated through creative activities like art and music.
Dr. Sam Gandy, Associate Director, Mount Sinai Alzheimer's Disease Research Center, NYC

The hippocampus[3] is affected, but the amygdala seems to be intact because individuals with Alzheimer's disease can express emotion. The amygdala is an almond shaped nucleus deep in the brain and it is very important in the expression and control of emotions.
Dr. Avertano Noronha, Neurologist, University of Chicago

The existing medications that are out there only give a little bit of symptomatic relief for a temporary period of time and with only some patients.
Dr. Robert Stern, Associate Professor of Neurology, Boston University

You know many people are confused about the difference between normal aging and the disease we call Alzheimer's disease. And it turns out that many people can age normally into very advanced age without losing their ability to think and remember so we know it's a disease. We know it doesn't have to happen, and in fact we now define it as a disease which has very specific pathology.
Dr. Robert Green, Associate Director for Research, Genetic Medicine, Brigham and Women's Hospital and Harvard Medical School

We are probably going to develop treatments to slow it down, but we're probably not going to have treatments to prevent it for some time, so in a way what we're going to have is more and more people living longer with Alzheimer's disease and a huge increase in the number of people living with the disease. So I think society has to think about that and to think about how are we going to deal with the epidemic of patients who have the disease.
Dr. Robert Green, Associate Director for Research, Genetic Medicine, Brigham and Women's Hospital and Harvard Medical School

---

3   The hippocampus is important for learning and short-term memory. This part of the brain is thought to be the site where short-term memories are converted into long-term memories for storage in other brain areas. (National Institute on Aging. *Alzheimer's Disease: Unraveling the Mystery.* 2008. p. 12)

The Effect of Alzheimer's Disease on the Individual

With the decline of cognitive skills, people with Alzheimer's usually lose self-confidence. They're afraid of their limitations and their loved ones stop involving them. Their daily activities diminish and progressively they become withdrawn. Alzheimer's reaches people from all walks of life, such as President Ronald Reagan, statesman Sargent Shriver, and actress Rita Hayworth, who was diagnosed with Alzheimer's in her 50's.
Olivia de Havilland, Narrator

The Effect of Creative Activities on People with Alzheimer's Disease

My mother always loved art…and in early to middle stages of Alzheimer's she decided that she wanted to paint. She loved oil, she loved the texture of oil. So she painted, and I think it brought her a peace of mind and it helped her to relax.
Yasmin Aga Khan, daughter of actress Rita Hayworth

What medicine has come to be impressed by is the therapeutic potential of the use of art and creative engagement as well as the impact on just contributions to the culture and feeling good and well being which are extremely important in their own right.
Dr. Gene Cohen, Director, Center on Aging, Health, and Humanities, George Washington University

Our goal is for people to use every skill they've got as long as they have it and to support this person's sense of well-being throughout the course of the illness. We connect with the person, with the human being that has that illness. They're not defined by their illness. They're defined by their personhood and who they are as a human being. When someone's painting a picture, that's using a motor skill. If someone if peeling a peach to make a pie, that's using a motor skill. And those skills and those experiences can help the person access memory using a different route than just asking the person directly.
Jane Stansell, Director, Alzheimer Family Care Center, Chicago

This is the first time I've ever seen her engaged in an art project. It's not something that she's ever done throughout her life and to see the concentration and the peace that being involved in a project like this evokes in her, knowing the kinds of transitions that she's been making over the last few years and to see the calm emanating from her soul at this moment is very, very rewarding and to look around at all the residents that we know and love and to see that kind of response is so meaningful.
Linda Stevenson, daughter of an Alzheimer's patient

I'm trying to help and support the person in artistic ways. It's a question of letting the sense emerge, and trying to reinsert that shape or color into the artwork which means maybe letting the person create an imaginary story sometimes with biographical references. But to reinsert its production into something that makes sense to the person and in particular of which he or she is the author—I think what I'm essentially doing is based on this idea of person and author. I'm not trying to confront or transform the condition resulting from the disease, but to find the bond that is possible with this person and the potential and individuality. So most of the time I think it's calling on physical sensations or body memory.
Patrick Laurin, Artist and Art Therapist, France Alzheimer's Center

The creative arts are a doorway. Once that doorway is opened and the caring proper knowledgeable stimulus delivered by a facilitator who understands the wonderful power of creative arts, once that stimulus is delivered to that person through that doorway, wonderful worlds open up. We know that they take in color, form, shape, and they process it in some way that is real, that is in the moment, and it translates in an Alzheimer's person's brain to have some meaning. The creative arts are an avenue to tap into a non-verbal emotional place in a person. When they're given paint, markers, any kind of media for art-making, and their hands are involved, and their muscles are involved, things are tapped in them that are genuine, and active and alive that don't get tapped

in our normal day social interaction, where we sit at the table and we make conversations over a meal or we read a newspaper and talk about the headlines of the day. So the creative arts bypass the limitations and they simply go to the strengths. People still have imagination intact all the way to the very, very end of their progressive disease.
Judy Holstein, Director, CJE Senior Life Day Center, Chicago

You can bring art to people with Alzheimer's, or you can bring them to art. A visit to a museum is a stimulating experience, one that seems to unlock emotions, speech, and memory even further, so much so that it becomes harder to recognize that they are affected by the disease.
Olivia de Havilland, Narrator

Visiting a museum or drawing or painting may not always engage every Alzheimer's resident. Caregivers and occupational therapists can then turn to a large spectrum of other activities to engage the person. These include music, singing, and dancing, story telling and poetry, memory workshop, taking care of pets, having physical activities, gardening, or simply cooking or baking a cake. A resident may not be fully engaged in a drawing workshop one day, but can be found the next day applauding enthusiastically at the circus when the horses appear onstage or when the acrobats start their performance.
Olivia de Havilland, Narrator

In spite of Alzheimer's, the essence of each person continues on, still ready to communicate, often through new paths, to touch and be touched, to love and be loved.
Olivia de Havilland, Narrator

Societal Views of Alzheimer's Disease

People are always surprised. They say I saw that group that was with you and it doesn't seem like they have Alzheimer's, it doesn't seem like they have dementia. The reason why you see the person and

not the disease is because you're not relying on short-term memory. Short-tem memory is completely irrelevant when you're enjoying a masterpiece, or you're listening to a symphony, you're listening to something from Bach, so what happens is you get the person. The person comes to the forefront, and not a bunch of symptoms.
Sean Caulfield, Creative Director, Artists for Alzheimer's (ARTZ)

If I help that person paint, they'll remember better. If I help that person drum, that person will be more present. If I help that person do crochet, that person will be more present. We have to help the families understand that the person is still there—then the families treat them with greater respect, greater dignity, and the people themselves have a sense of who they are, which is a magnificent thing to see.
John Zeisel, President Hearthstone Alzheimer's Foundation

The State of Alzheimer's Care Today

Of the 6 million people living with Alzheimer's disease in north America and of the 7 million in Europe, less than 15 percent are engaged in physical therapies, occupational therapies, or creative activities.
Olivia de Havilland, Narrator

Nursing homes in America are still quite dreadful. Only one of 10 nursing homes actually meet basic federal standards with respect to the adequate staffing, so the idea of staff really having the time to spend time with their patients devoted to enriching their lives is very unlikely, unfortunately. We're talking about one and a half million people in 15,000 nursing homes. Again to repeat, only one in 10 meet basic federal standards with respect to personnel. So we're going to have to change all that if we're going to make use of the role of the arts and the role of memory and other prospects of enlivening the lives of those with dementia.
Dr. Robert Butler, Founding Director, National Institute on Aging

13 References and Resources
Assistance for Alzheimer's Patients, Their Families, and Their Caregivers

Dorothy Seman, R.N., M.S. and Berna G. Huebner

There is a growing medical and popular literature on Alzheimer's disease and other memory disorders and a gradually increasing literature on art therapy related to these conditions. Websites for many organizations can provide access to information and relationships. All of this can provide much support for persons who are facing the sometimes terrifying advent of memory loss and who are interested in exploring creative engagement as a means of ameliorating some of its effects. The editors present the following selective list of resources as a beginning point for all those who are searching for help.

Websites

The Hilgos Foundation
www.hilgos.org
> This site gives the visitor the opportunity to enter the world of an artist whose life and legacy gave rise to this project, in its many forms: Hilda's determined spirit, her persona, comes through her paintings. That insistence on continuing to create has taught others that we must not dismiss or underestimate what lies just below the surface. Hilda's gift to us of color and brushstroke and geometric forms ... combine with vistas of open waters and conveyances ....floating alone but near to one another, unique but sharing common space. These announce

that despite some diminishments of aging there often remains exuberance and an insistence on living. We too are invited to set sail and to find the wind … or create the wind of change. Living life richly at the far end of the waters often requires some light and lighthouse keeper… someone to beckon us home, to signal for us if we should for a moment have lost our way.

Copies of the Hilgos paintings appearing in this book are available for sale through the Hilgos Foundation website.

Alzheimer's Association
www.alz.org

This site is an entry point that can guide families throughout the course of the journey with Alzheimer's disease. It is a roadmap that guides your search for virtually any question that relates to Alzheimer's care. There is information about the disease process, or can link to resources, for diagnosis, care centers and services you or your family member may need. Provides information about Alzheimer's in many languages other than English. An international conference is held annually. See www.alz.org/AAIC.

USAgainstAlzheimer's
www.usagainstalzheimers.org

USAgainstAlzheimer's is a national advocacy campaign and independent advocacy network committed to stopping Alzheimer's by 2020.

Family Caregiver Alliance
www.caregiver.org

This organization has a long tradition of helping caregivers who are caring for individuals with special needs. It does focus on Alzheimer's specifically. It helps family caregivers understand how to be an advocate for their family member, and how to identify what services are needed to keep the family unit in balance. It provides a variety of practical, and focused how-to guides to obtain needed help in the home or resolve issues that arise with other family members, employers, and health care providers.

The Hartford Insurance
www.thehartford.com/alzheimers/

Provides guidance to help the reader assess when driving becomes a risk for the person with Alzheimer's and others; and offers useful approaches to weighing options and making tough decisions. The material provides practical suggestions about how to balance sensitivity and safety. Suggests ways to help smooth the transitions that will be necessary as the disease progresses.

Alzheimer's Disease Education & Referral Center
www.nia.nih.gov/Alzheimers/ResearchInformation/ResearchCenters/

This link takes you to the federal government website that can help you locate the federally funded Alzheimer's research center that is most convenient for you. These centers can provide a thorough evaluation and diagnosis. They often provide support groups and identify agencies that provide a range of services that might be needed over time. Most centers provide educational programs on Alzheimer's. If the travel distance is too great, the staff will help you identify local medical centers closer to you that are affiliated with universities. They can help match your needs with a medical center that has specialized staff or programs, including the opportunity to participate in research studies.

Everyday Health
www.everydayhealth.com

This website carried an extended interview with Dr. John Zeisel, the author of *I'm Still Here* (see the Books section), and artist Phyllis Beinart. The interview is at www.everydayhealth.com/alzheimers/webcasts/art-therapy-for-alzheimers-and-dementia.aspx.

Artists for Alzheimer's (ARTZ)
www.artistsforalzheimers.org

ARTZ is an initiative of the Hearthstone Alzheimer's Foundation that uses art to enrich the cultural life or people afflicted with Alzheimer's disease.

National Association of Professional Geriatric Care Managers
www.caremanager.org

This organization can help family caregivers locate a geriatric care manager in the community where a family member lives. They can provide a wide array of services on a fee for service basis. This includes making health care appointments, arranging transportation and accompanying person to appointments; arranging and conducting interviews for in-home help, companions, or community services. This individual can often help construct an overall plan of care that includes medical care and treatment as well as assistance that helps foster quality of life while accommodating changing needs.

Eldercare Locator
www.eldercare.gov

The Eldercare Locator is a public service of the U.S. Administration on Aging. It is a first step to finding resources for older adults in any U.S. community. Using either the website or making a phone call can help you get the help you need. You can get an overview of potential kinds of services that might be available to you and your family. If you already know what you are looking for, this resource may help you locate specific programs or services in your community

You can find local information resources by following the directions on the website or calling 1-800-677-1116. Visit the *Resources* section of Eldercare.gov to learn about additional federal and national information sources.

Dementia Advocacy and Support Network
www.dasninternational.org/

Men and women diagnosed with Alzheimer's and other forms of dementia have created an online support system called the Dementia Advocacy and Support Network. Some members have written books that describe what helps them cope. There are links to these books on this site. A common theme is the importance of friends and family helping them to maintain continuity with their identity, relationships and activities as their memory or planning interrupts the steps needed to complete activities that give them comfort and pleasure.

Center on Age and Community
www.ageandcommunity.org

This is the website of the Center on Age and Community of the University of Wisconsin, Milwaukee. Its Director, Dr. Anne Basting, is also Associate Professor of Theater Arts (see the Books section). The Center has published, among other works, *ArtCare*, a manual profiling "a person-centered, creative engagement artist in residency program," and *TimeSlips Training Manual*, a guide to "a storytelling technique that encourages people with memory loss to exercise their imagination and creativity." (See reference by Dr. Cohen in Chapter 2.)

The Remembering Site
www.therememberingsite.org/

The Remembering Site makes it easy for anyone, anywhere to write and publish their life story and add to it as life unfolds. Everyone can leave family treasures made of words. The evocative questions on The Remembering Site make this as easy as possible for you. You will also have the opportunity to print quality paperback or hardback copies of your memoir to share.

Cure Alzheimer's Fund
www.curealz.org

This site targets breakthrough research.

Alzheimer's Disease International (ADI)
www.alz.co.uk

> The global Voice on Dementia—an umbrella organization of national Alzheimer Associations around the world.

Alzheimer's Drug Discovery Foundation (ADDF)
www.alzdiscovery.org

> Drug discovery research defines ADDF and their mission. Accelerating new drugs to prevent, treat and ultimately cure Alzheimer's Disease is their goal.

National Center for Creative Aging (NCCA)
www.creativeaging.org

> The National Center for Creative Aging is dedicated to fostering an understanding of the vital relationship between creative expression and the quality of life of older people. Creative expression is important for older people of all cultures and ethnic backgrounds, regardless of economic status, age, or level of physical, emotional, or cognitive functioning.

The MoMA Alzheimer's Project
www.MoMA.org/meetme

> The MoMA Alzheimer's Project is the nationwide expansion of MoMA's art and dementia programs, including Meet Me at MoMA, the Museum's outreach program for individuals living with Alzheimer's disease and their caregivers.

Arts for the Aging, Inc. (AFTA)
www.aftaarts.com

> AFTA provides artistic services to impaired seniors in day care centers and not-for-profit nursing homes in the metropolitan Washington area.

Society for Arts in Healthcare (SAH)
www.thesah.org

> The Society for the Arts in Healthcare is dedicated to advancing arts as integral to healthcare.

Alzheimer's Foundation (AFA)
www.alzfdn.org
>AFA helps provide care to Americans affected by Alzheimer's disease and other related illnesses. AFA and its member organizations offer education and hands-on services that can improve quality of life for individuals with the disease and their families.

Books

"I Remember Better When I Paint" Resource Book
>Download from www.hilgos.org.
>Lists medical and educational centers, nursing homes and residences, museums, films, books, and other helpful resources.

The Creative Age: Awakening Human Potential in the Second Half of Life
>Gene D. Cohen, M.D., Ph.D., Avon Books, New York, 2000.

>An introduction to the potential opportunities for creativity in older people, by one of the early leaders in geriatrics and geriatric research.

The Stages of Age: Performing Age in Contemporary American Culture
>Anne D. Basting, Ph.D., University of Michigan Press, Ann Arbor, 1998.

Dementia Reconsidered: The Person Comes First
>T. M. Kitwood, Open University Press, Buckingham, United Kingdom, 1997

The Person with Alzheimer's Disease: Pathways to Understanding the Experience
>Edited by Phyllis Braudy Harris, Johns Hopkins University Press, Baltimore, 2002

>Some chapters may be equally helpful for family caregivers and staff who work in programs that serve people with Alzheimer's. The strength of this book is the way it portrays the resilience of those living with Alzheimer's. Chapters explore how the human spirit can be preserved by nurturing and joyful relationships

that arise in the course shared self expression. The challenges and difficulties of dementia are not ignored but accepted. There are descriptions of volunteer programs and art therapy groups that focus on creating a fabric of interactions that allow self expression that reaches surprising depths.

A Dignified Life: The Best Friends Approach to Alzheimer's Care, A Guide for Family Caregivers
Virginia Bell & David Troxel, Health Communications Press, Deerfield Beach Florida, 2003

These authors have a very conversational reading style. They explore ways to re-evaluate how their relationship with someone with dementia has changed as a result of the diagnosis. They explore some interactions that create stressful interaction. Drawing on their experience with many families, they offer innovative ways to identify "trigger points" and then describe ways to minimize or avoid these. They focus on planning out family focused activities that support abilities and do not have expectations that exceed the persons abilities.

The Alzheimer's Health Care Handbook: How to Get the Best Medical Care for Your Relative with Alzheimer's disease, in and out of the Hospital.
Mary S. Mittelman, D.P.H, and C. Epstein; Avalon Publishing Group, Inc., New York, 2003.

Learning to Speak Alzheimer's
Joanne Koenig Coste, Houghton Mifflin Company, Boston, 2004

This book helps caregivers to maintain the perspective that if we listen and observe attentively family can often sustain meaningful and satisfying relationships. She helps family focus on the needs of person with Alzheimer's and how small adaptations ions can help

The Mature Mind – The Positive Power of the Aging Brain
Gene D. Cohen, M.D., Ph.D., Basic Books, New York, 2005

An overview of some of the implications of what the author, one of the early leaders in aging research, calls the "big news":

"the brain is far more flexible and adaptable than once thought. . . . it can grow entirely new brain cells." The two appendices contain valuable resource lists of relevant literature and other resources for those interested in creativity and aging.

Getting to Know the Life Stories of Older Adults: Activities for Building Relationships
Kathy Laurenhue, Health Professions Press, Baltimore, 2007

This reference provides a structure of questions, organized by topic areas that can help draw out memories of meaningful activities. It can be used to jump start conversation about art and music and theater that elicit fond memories. Pictures help to establish a sense of time and place that can re-kindle memories, making you feel more alive and connected to the others and to the world around you.

I'm Still Here
John Zeisel, Ph.D., The Penguin Group, New York, 2009

With chapters on the Alzheimer's brain, visual art and Alzheimer's and the dramatic arts, this book outlines a number of strategies for relating to the person who remains within the Alzheimer's patient.

Jan's Story: Love Lost to the Long Goodbye of Alzheimer's
Barry Petersen, Behler Publications, 2010.

A veteran television news correspondent tells a moving personal story of coping with early onset Alzheimer's disease. See also www.barrypetersen.com.

I Love You…Who Are You? Loving and Caring for a Parent with Alzheimer's
Patti Kerr, Along the Way Press, 2010.

The author, whose mother and grandmother had Alzheimer's, interviews family members who cared for a loved one with the disease. See also www.pattikerr.com

Forget Memory: Creating Better Lives for People with Dementia
Anne D. Basting, Ph.D., The Johns Hopkins University Press, Baltimore, 2009

This book is by the director of the Center for Age and Community at the University of Wisconsin, Milwaukee.

Still Alice
Lisa Genova, Pocket Books, New York, 2009

A fictional story of a Harvard psychology professor who is diagnosed with early onset Alzheimer's. It contains valuable information about Alzheimer's Disease.

Passages in Caregiving
Gail Sheehy, Harper-Collins, New York, 2010

Ms. Sheehy writes about her own caregiving experience and discusses the eight stages of caregiving from "Shock and Mobilization" to "The Long Good-Bye." She covers the challenges and rewards inherent in caregiving, the U.S. health care system, and the patient's need to be part of the decision making process.

Games

Making Memories Together
Gene D. Cohen, M.D., Ph.D., Genco International, Inc.

This award-winning noncompetitive board game designed by Dr. Gene Cohen is for persons with major memory disorders, such as Alzheimer's disease. Families are instructed on how to create individualized Memory Cards that help tap into pockets of preserved memories for the memory impaired individual, thereby improving the quality of visits. It is available from www.genco-games.com/making-memories.html

Puzzle With Me
Jane Snyder, Creater and CEO, Puzzle with Me, Inc.

Jigsaw puzzles to help caregivers and people with dementia communicate. They are available from www.puzzlewithme.com.

Films and Plays

I Remember Better When I Paint

> Eric Ellena and Berna Huebner, Co-Directors. French Connection Films and the Hilgos Foundation, 2009, available on Amazon.com. Trailer at <u>irememberbetterwhenipaint.com</u>.

> This groundbreaking documentary shows how the creative arts can change the quality of life for people with Alzheimer's. Filmed in America and Europe, it shows Alzheimer's patients focusing and reconnecting as they paint at their homes and care facilities and visit the Louvre in Paris, the Art Institute in Chicago, the Phillips Collection in Washington, DC, and the Big Apple Circus in New York. The film is narrated by Olivia de Havilland and features Yasmin Aga Khan, president of Alzheimer's Disease International and daughter of Rita Hayworth, who had Alzheimer's and painted. It includes interviews with renowned neurologists who explain how creative activities engage areas of the brain that are not damaged by the disease and thus help reawaken a sense of personality, identity, and dignity. The extended DVD version includes seven Bonus Features of new creative therapies for those with memory impairment.

I Remember Better When I Paint (Alzheimer's Play)

> This seven-minute play, created by the Hilgos Foundation, is for young students and is based on the concept that children will respond to a story if they participate in telling it. Children read from a script that dramatizes the narrative of Hilgos and the students who painted with her. The play can be used to open a longer discussion in classrooms, in day care centers, in assisted living facilities, and with community groups who are interested in these issues. It can be seen at <u>www.youtube.com/watch?v=iy1_IkAEN8Y</u>.

Painting in Twilight: An Artist's Escape from Alzheimer's

> Features the art of Lester Potts, who learned to express his thoughts and feelings through art after being diagnosed with

Alzheimer's in his 70s. Shown on YouTube and produced for UAB Magazine (University of Alabama at Birmingham) by The Periodicals Group. For more information, see Cognitive Dynamics (www.cognitivedynamics.org/).

Recent Research

Non-Pharmacological Therapies For Alzheimer's Disease Need Be Made Widely Available - Study

22 scientists have published a study they say provides clear evidence about the effectiveness of Non-pharmacological Therapies in Alzheimer's disease. A cure for Alzheimer's is not in sight and available drugs have worthwhile but limited benefits. They say approaches such as cognitive stimulation and physical exercise can improve cognitive function, mood and behavior symptoms of people with dementia. For more information, see www.science20.com/news_articles/ nonpharmacological_therapies_alzheimers_disease_need_be_ made_widely_available_study

Endorsements for
I Remember Better When I Paint

Powerful insights on an exploding epidemic.
Richard Reeves, Author and Journalist

This is an inspirational story of an artist who finally was able to paint again. The idea is that the creative arts can help people who have Alzheimer's now. They open a pathway to the nonverbal emotional place in the person.
Yasmin Aga Khan, President, Alzheimer's Disease International, Daughter of actress Rita Hayworth

...illuminates a breakthrough in connecting to people with Alzheimer's—through art. It's a story that needs to be passed on to every caregiver who fears that Alzheimer's has robbed the mind and soul of a beloved, forever.
Gail Sheehy, Author and Journalist

...a real message of hope and an important contribution to changing the way people look at Alzheimer's Disease.
Marc Wortmann, CEO, Alzheimer's Disease International

Alzheimer's typically hits memory areas of the brain early while sparing areas responsible for creativity. Art and music are perfect modalities for stimulating these creativity areas. This strategy is also an effective way to relieve agitation without sedating drugs. I Remember Better When I Paint presents a comprehensive and compelling account of how the arts can help change the quality of life for people with memory impairment.
Dr. Sam Gandy, Associate Director, Mount Sinai Alzheimer's Disease Research Center, NYC

I Remember Better When I Paint points the way as we fight for the dignity for all those with Alzheimer's and dementia, seeking to unravel the mystery of how to connect with those who cannot communicate as they have in the past. These are our parents, our spouses, our friends—we must find new and creative ways to express our love and to permit them to communicate their love for life and for us.
Trish and George Vradenburg co-founders of USAgainstAlzheimer's

Engagement throughout the course of Alzheimer's is important for the quality of life for the person with the disease. Art programs offer a unique opportunity for people to express themselves, particularly those whose disease has progressed to the point of limited communication. Participating in art or other reminiscence therapies can help people with Alzheimer's and other dementias connect and relate to their past and build bridges to present interactions.
Beth Kallmyer, LCSW, Senior Director, Constituent Services, Alzheimer's Association

I Remember Better When I Paint is a must-read for anyone involved with the care of individuals with Alzheimer's disease (AD), including professionals and family members. The book exquisitely demonstrates the power of the arts in the treatment of those afflicted with this disease. Although much of the brain progressively deteriorates, some of the last areas to be hurt in AD are those involved with the emotional responses to the arts. This book, through its poignant and touching stories, clearly shows that there are so many important things we can all do to improve the quality of life of those with Alzheimer's.
Dr. Robert A. Stern, Professor of Neurology and Neurosurgery; Director, Alzheimer's Disease Center Clinical Core, Boston University School of Medicine

This remarkable work embraces contemporary and life-affirming ideas concerning how to bring out the best in the person with Alzheimer's disease or other dementia. I admire the ambition behind this book, demonstrating how creativity remains, even when memory has diminished. The book will inspire us all to focus on strengths instead of losses. A great resource for family and professional caregivers.

David Troxel, MPH, Co-Author, The Best Friends Approach to Alzheimer's Care
Past Executive Director, Alzheimer's Association, Santa Barbara, CA

I Remember When I Paint shows the intersection of the arts and medicine and how the creative arts help people with Alzheimer's. As a practicing creative arts therapist, I have witnessed the transformations that can take place. Physicians provide explanations based on brain science; art therapists provide clinical explanations; the artists themselves provide the greatest proof of all: their heightened pride and joy that results from art experiences. I Remember Better When I Paint leaves us with new understanding of the helpfulness of creative arts for people with Alzheimer's.

Judy Holstein, MS, LPC, RDT/BCT, Director, Adult Day Services, CJE SeniorLife, Chicago, Illinois

Printed in Great Britain
by Amazon.co.uk, Ltd.,
Marston Gate.